I dedicate this book to my twin sister, Rhonda Flagstad, who inspired me to live a healthier, fitter life!

THE SSASS WORKOUT
Sixty Second ASS

Sixty Seconds a Day to Firm, Trim, Tone Your ASS (AKA, Bum or Tush) For a Sexy Rear-End!

Published by MajorVision International

2017

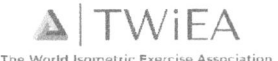

The World Isometric Exercise Association

Approved by The World Isometric Exercise Association

www.HelenRenee.com – www.BrianSterlingVete.com

Contents

www.HelenRenee.com – www.BrianSterlingVete.com

Chapter 1: Important General Safety and Health Guidelines

This disclaimer applies to all content contained within or associated with this book, including but not limited to: books, courses, articles, publications of any kind, videos, associated websites, recommendations, suggestions, coaching, and any advice whether written, digital, verbal, or otherwise, created or delivered by Brian Sterling-Vete and Helen Renée Wuorio, who are the copyright holders, creators, instructors, and originators of the material herein.

Medical Approval Required

You must not undertake any exercise programme, course, or dietary change referenced in this book or related materials without first obtaining full approval from a qualified medical doctor.

Only your doctor is able to determine your suitability for the physical activities or dietary practices described, particularly if you have any known or suspected medical conditions, are pregnant, or have other significant health concerns.

You are strongly advised to present all relevant content from this book, including any associated videos, audio material, or online content, to your doctor for review and to obtain their written or verbal approval prior to beginning any exercise or diet plan.

Not a Substitute for Personalised Professional Advice

The exercises, plans, recommendations, and suggestions provided are intended solely as general reference material. They are not tailored to individual circumstances and do not constitute professional, personalised medical or fitness advice. They must not be relied upon as a replacement for a qualified personal trainer, fitness coach, dietitian, or medical professional. This material is not intended for use by children, and all exercise equipment should be kept out of reach of minors.

Exercise Caution and Equipment Safety

You must always exercise caution and avoid overexertion. If you experience any pain, discomfort, shortness of breath, chest pain, irregular heartbeat, faintness, dizziness, nausea, or any other concerning symptom, stop exercising immediately and seek medical assistance without delay.

Before each use, you must thoroughly inspect all exercise equipment—whether purpose-made or improvised—as well as any doorways, frames, floors, benches, chairs, or furniture used for exercising. Equipment should only be used if it is in proper working order, free from visible damage or wear, and securely positioned to avoid injury.

Always take care when transitioning into or out of exercise positions, particularly when moving to and from the floor or using any surfaces or objects for support.

Limitation of Liability

Neither Brian Sterling-Vete nor Helen Renée Wuorio, nor any person, company, or organisation associated with them, accepts any liability for injury, loss, harm, illness, damage to property, or any other adverse outcome—whether direct or indirect—arising from the use of any information, recommendations, exercises, or materials contained in this book or any related content, including websites and videos.

Further Guidance

For further general health and fitness information, we recommend consulting reputable sources such as:

The National Health Service (UK): https://www.nhs.uk/Livewell/fitness/pages/physical-activity-guidelines-for-adults.aspx

The Mayo Clinic (USA): https://www.mayoclinic.org/healthy-lifestyle

Chapter 2: Introduction

Let me start by telling you what The SSASS™ Workout means. **SSASS™ – Sixty Seconds** to a better **ASS,** The **S**ixty **S**econd **ASS** Workout or **SSASS™**! You will complete six exercises for 10 seconds each. A total of 60 seconds each day. It is as simple as that. I wanted to create a workout that is super effective and super-fast to lift and tone up our behinds.

I know that time is the biggest excuse people have nowadays for not exercising regularly. With our busy lives with work, school, and family commitments, comparatively few of us have the time to go to the gym and exercise as often as we would prefer. Therefore, I created the SSASS™ Workout, a highly intense, super-effective workout that is equal to 15 minutes of non-stop training in a gym. I am sure everybody can spare 60 seconds a day. (If you cannot, then you are not ready to transform your body yet!)

The other big complaint I hear from women all the time is that sitting at a desk all day or just not working out anymore, they have lost their ass, literally. Apologies for those offended by the word "ass" - bum, booty, butt, rear-end, behind, arse, or whatever else you want to call it; the truth is as we age, our backside gets flabby and saggy. I believe that everyone, no matter what their age, would like to lift, tone up and tighten the rear end.

The SSASS™ Workout will be equally effective for the advanced athlete as well. Even if you already have a great bum, you want to maintain those sexy curves, and it is not always easy to get to the gym. This is the perfect exercise to complete in a hotel room, whether on vacation or travelling for business. The SSASS™ Workout is also designed with time, ease of use and flexibility in mind so that you can enjoy and benefit from a professional-level workout virtually anywhere.

We have received positive testimonials and useful feedback from many other people in different countries who were some of our early followers and enthusiasts of the system, thanks to our The 70 Second Difference™ book.

With the ISOfitness™ exercise system and The SSASS™ Workout, the choice of where and when you exercise is always *your* choice. It is never a choice imposed on you due to the traditional confines and restrictions of less efficient ways of exercising, which require heavy and bulky equipment. This is true Fitness on the Move™.

Chapter 3: Exercise Science Overview

In this chapter, we will provide a user-friendly overview of exercise science and discuss the features and benefits of various exercise techniques and concepts. For those who want more in-depth information about the science of isometric exercise and health and fitness in general, we suggest that you also read our books The ISOmetric Bible™ and The 70 Second Difference™. Both are available on Amazon.

Walking as Exercise

Walking is a vastly underrated form of exercise; even a short, regular daily walk can yield tremendous health benefits. In recent years, several notable studies have been performed on the health-related benefits of walking and how walking can even help prevent many serious diseases and illnesses.

In the journal Healthy Heart for Life!, Dr Martha Grogan of the Mayo Clinic in Rochester, Minnesota, said that research indicates that walking for just 10 minutes a day can halve one's risk of having a heart attack. She also noted that a sedentary lifestyle increases the risk of a heart attack almost as much as smoking does.

Therefore, given that golf typically involves walking far longer than just 10 minutes a day, even golfers are dramatically cutting their risk of a heart attack while simultaneously having fun. Whereas Nordic Walkers and Trekkers naturally gain even greater health-related benefits due to the greater distances they walk.

In Great Britain, the NHS research indicates the same as the Mayo Clinic research. After the results of an extensive international study were published, the National Health Service highly recommends walking as an excellent form of exercise that helps to prevent several serious illnesses and diseases.

Other studies focused on adults with a high risk of type 2 diabetes and heart disease. Research has found that an additional 2,000 steps per day lowered the risk of experiencing a cardiac issue by up to 10% for this group of people. Furthermore, continuing research indicated that for every additional 2,000 steps per day that were taken, the risk was further reduced by 8%. The research was carried out by teams from the NIHR Leicester-Loughborough Diet, Lifestyle, and Physical Activity Biomedical Research Unit, the University of Leicester, and Duke University School of Medicine in the USA. They also collaborated with other researchers from universities and institutes around the world. The results were published in the medical journal The Lancet.

Research indicates that two and a half hours of walking each week can also help to reduce the risk of contracting seven types of cancer. The research suggested that it reduced the risk of kidney cancer in both sexes by 11 per cent and by 17 per cent if the length of time spent walking/taking moderate exercise was increased to five hours per week. The research also suggested that two and a half hours of walking each week could reduce the risk of contracting breast cancer by 5%, and by 10% for five hours of walking per week. Women were up to 18% less likely to get cancer of the womb, both sexes were less likely to get

15

non-Hodgkin's lymphoma, up to 19 per cent less likely to contract myeloma, and men were up to 14% less likely to get colon cancer. The details of the study were published in the Journal of Clinical Oncology.

Walking Vs Running as a Fat Burner

Walking and running are both excellent ways to get fitter, burn calories, tone up, and promote weight loss. There are different and distinct benefits to each, which we will briefly touch on. Running burns more calories than walking does. However, walking burns more fat than running does. So, it is a trade-off, especially since walking more will increase your N.E.A.T. factor. We will explain more about N.E.A.T. in the next section.

When exercising at a lower intensity, fat is used as the body's primary fuel. When you shift gears and increase the pace from walking to running, your body burns more carbohydrates as fuel.

However, it does not matter too much whether you are burning body fat or carbohydrates as the primary fuel. What is important is that you burn the most calories possible during your exercise session and stimulate a long-term increase in your Base Metabolic Rate. Therefore, even though walking may burn more stored fat as fuel, running will still burn more overall calories.

Another important factor to consider when comparing the differences between walking and running is the risk of injury. Running carries more risk of injury than walking, so the choice is yours.

Walking, General Activity and N.E.A.T. - Non-Exercise Activity Thermogenesis

The acronym N.E.A.T. is becoming increasingly discussed in relation to weight control, body fat, and exercise. The N.E.A.T. acronym stands for Non-Exercise Activity Thermogenesis, and it comes from Dr James Levine's research into how we expend calories. In simple terms, it means: "burning calories through daily life, and not through exercise," and in the simplest terms, it means that people who are active and move around a lot burn more calories and tend to be slimmer than people who do not.

There are two basic ways in which we burn calories. One is while we exercise, and the other is through the general activities of daily living. The key question is: "Which, if any, is more important to weight loss, and what are the levels of body fat that we carry?" According to Dr Levine, it is the N.E.A.T. that appears to be far more important for calorie burning than dedicated exercise time. Dr Levine's research also led to the phrase "Being Active Naturally" becoming more commonly used.

Providing that you exercise good judgment in your food choices and the macros around proper portion control, in addition to your regular exercise routine, just being a little more active in everyday life will make a huge difference in terms of weight control and overall body fat levels.

In our opinion, N.E.A.T. alone is not a great panacea when it comes to losing weight and staying slim. After all, when people are stressed and mentally fatigued because of a tough workday, it is not always easy to opt for the most sensible food choices, nor is it likely that you will want to go out and do something active to increase your daily movement factor. However, N.E.A.T. is certainly something to be factored into your overall lifestyle because it makes a significant difference to your overall appearance and fitness levels.

The Basic Types of Resistance Exercise

All muscle training falls into two or three specific categories, depending on how you break them down. In the most basic form, there are two types: contraction with or without movement. Breaking them down a step further, there become three categories, with one being isotonic, another isokinetic, and last but certainly not least, isometric.

Isotonic training is all about movement, with muscle shortening and lengthening during the lifting and lowering phases of the exercise. We know that the isotonic category can be broken down further into three parts. One part is the concentric contraction, which is the lifting phase of an exercise when the muscles shorten. Another is the eccentric phase, the lowering part of an exercise when the muscles lengthen.

Lastly, the isotonic category includes the isokinetic contraction. In this contraction, the muscle changes in length during both the concentric and eccentric phases; however, the velocity remains constant no matter how much force is applied during the exercises.

Then comes the isometric category. With an isometric exercise, there is no movement whatsoever. To help you envision this, I will take a random weight training or freehand callisthenic exercise, such as a chest press, because it can be performed either with movement OR without movement as an isometric exercise.

For example, a barbell, a machine, or your bodyweight can be lifted and lowered to perform an exercise such as a barbell curl. This is called isotonic exercise, callisthenics, or simply exercise with movement.

To perform the same or similar exercise isometrically, you would attempt to perform the same or similar biomechanically correct actions of a barbell curl. However, at a certain point, or points if multiple exercise points were being used, the curling movement would stop because an immovable object point had been reached.

At that point or points, you would apply an increasing level of force until you reach the desired target level as you attempt to perform the curling exercise against the immovable object.

At the desired isometric exercise point, a constant force is applied against the immovable object for 7 seconds, which is the optimum isometric exercise time. The ideal basic isometric exercise point for general exercise is roughly at the mid-point when your muscles reach a stalemate working against each other or an immovable object. This is called a Standard isometric Contraction.

The harder you engage your muscles as you try to break the stalemate by lifting, pushing, or pulling, the stronger your muscles become. In doing so, you engage many more muscle fibres than normal as you attempt to move the immovable object and perform the curling exercise action.

Doors, desks, chairs, walls, and many other everyday items can serve as immovable objects. However, the simplest and most accessible immovable object is often yourself, making isometric exercise a convenient and empowering choice.

Isometric Overview

As you now know, isometric exercise does not involve any movement. Instead, the joint angle and the muscle length do not change during contraction. You also now know that 7 seconds is regarded as the optimum time to perform an isometric exercise.

However, almost everyone tends to count the exercise elapsed time much faster than the real elapsed time when exercising. This means that it is easy not to reach the magic 7 seconds of the optimum isometric exercise time. Therefore, we always suggest aiming to perform the exercise for 10 seconds to ensure that the 7-second target is always reached, even when under the stress of intense exercise.

Isometric exercise has been extensively scientifically researched and repeatedly proven to be a highly effective method for building strength and muscle. It is one of the most thoroughly researched exercise systems despite being one of the most misunderstood. This is likely due to fear, professional ignorance, and financial reasons, but the evidence of its effectiveness is undeniable.

The isometric exercise system can use several different techniques. Most of these techniques are highly advanced and intended for competitive athletes, martial arts practitioners, strength athletes, and bodybuilders. Therefore, they are not appropriate for a general isometric exercise session for the average person who simply wants to get stronger and fitter.

However, purely out of interest, I will list them here in case any fitness enthusiasts, athletes, or bodybuilders read this book and wish to try them. They are described in greater detail in our book called The Isometric Bible, which is available on Amazon and in good bookstores. The most common and advanced isometric exercise techniques include the following:

- Standard Isometric Contraction
- Yielding Isometric Contraction
- Maximum Duration Isometrics
- Oscillatory Isometrics
- Impact Absorption Isometrics
- Explosive Isometrics, AKA: Ballistic Isometrics
- Static-Dynamic Isometric
- Contrast Isometric
- Functional Isometrics
- TRISOmetrics™

More than enough isometric exercises can be performed without any equipment to allow a total body workout routine to be completed relatively easily. These will typically be self-resisting isometric exercises, which are excellent. However, by using only minimal readily available equipment such as walking poles, golf clubs, martial arts belts, climbing ropes, scuba diving webbing, weight belts, and broom handles, etc., it is possible to greatly expand the number of exercises that can be performed.

It is also perfectly possible to adapt and use other readily available items such as tow ropes, steel chains, towels, and commonly found immobile objects such as sturdy fixed barrier railings, solid walls, solid doors, door frames, or parked vehicles to perform a complete isometric exercise routine. Again, these are all excellent improvised exercise tools that allow an expanded range of highly effective isometric exercises to be performed.

Using improvised exercise tools can yield an unexpected additional benefit. This is because it allows one to focus more and apply greater concentration to each exercise. This is particularly useful for those who are either completely new to or are relatively new to the isometric exercise system. We will explain more about what these can be later in the book.

One of the things we love about both the isometric and self-resisted exercise systems is that as you get stronger through exercise, you can apply more force and intensity to your isometric or self-resisted exercises.

This, in turn, means that you can gradually increase the level of force and intensity you can safely apply to each exercise, which will mean that the results and benefits you receive will grow in a compound way through regular daily use. This is what we call a natural Adaptive Response™ mechanism, which is a useful aspect of our biology.

Isometric Exercise Science

Even until the mid-20th century, almost no scientific research had been performed on the benefits of isometric exercise. We also know that before the first serious scientific research study, people were trained isometrically by performing what we now call endurance isometrics.

Thankfully, isometric exercise has been thoroughly scientifically researched and proven for several decades. I would estimate that at least as much scientific research has been performed on it as on traditional resistance training.

The first major in-depth study into isometric exercise was performed at the world-famous Max Planck Institute in Dortmund, Germany. If you already have a reasonable knowledge of science, you will also know that the Max Planck Institute is a world-renowned centre of scientific excellence in many disciplines.

Between 1953 and 1958, one of the most extensive research studies was commissioned into isometric exercise science. Many consider these experiments to be the original gold standard of isometric exercise studies. The results were made widespread public knowledge in the resultant ground-breaking book, The Physiology of Strength, by Dr Theodor Hettinger, Research Fellow at the Max Planck Institute. During that 5-year research period, Dr Hettinger and Dr Muller performed a widely reported, reputed 5,500 experiments, although this figure is almost certainly apocryphal because they would have had to perform a minimum of three experiments a day, every day for five years.

Research suggests that the actual number of experiments performed by Hettinger and Muller was probably less than 50. However, many thousands of studies have almost certainly been completed at other institutions worldwide since then. These were conducted on male and female volunteers from all walks of life and at every level of strength, fitness, and athletic ability. Perhaps what surprised people the most was how dramatic and impressive the results were gained from performing isometric exercises. Also, because the same or similar results were easily repeatable, the data gained from the experiments was exceptionally reliable. The conclusion of the extensive studies proved beyond doubt the overall superiority of isometric exercise in building strength and muscle compared to traditional isotonic exercise methods. It also proved that the isometric system delivered these results much faster and with far less exercise than traditional resistance training.

Another extremely interesting result emerged from the experiments. This was because the optimum results were not produced by the length of time an isometric exercise was held, but by the correct level of force applied for a specific optimum time.

They found that performing only one daily isometric exercise for between 6 and 7 seconds and at only two-thirds of an individual's maximum effort could increase strength by an average of up to 5% per week. By any standards, strength gains of 5% in exchange for the expenditure of only 66%, or around two-thirds of an individual's maximum capacity, is an excellent result.

Perhaps even more amazingly, they discovered that after someone has performed a single 7-second training stimulus (exercise) per day, the muscle being exercised in that same position was no longer responsive to further gains. In other words, it did not matter how many more times you exercised the same muscle in the same position; there would be no further increase in muscle growth or strength. The only way to do this was to perform another isometric exercise at a different position, only the limb's ROM (Range Of Motion). The scientific data about this can be referenced on pages 28 to 31 of Dr Theodor Hettinger's book, "The Physiology of Strength."

In 2001, Nicolas Babault, PhD of the University of Burgundy, Dijon, France, led a team of scientists to research and examine how many muscle fibres were activated and how long they remained active during both traditional weight training and isometric training.

(The scientific research paper is published: Nicolas Babault, Michel Pousson, Yves Ballay, and Jacques Van Hoecke - Groupe Analyse du Mouvement, Unite´ de Formation et de Recherche Sciences et Techniques des Activite´s Physiques et Sportives, Universite´ de Bourgogne, BP 27877, 21078 Dijon Cedex, France.)

They discovered that when training intensely and in near-perfect style, the levels of muscle activation during repetitions of optimum maximal weight training were between 89.7% during the concentric contraction, or when lifting a weight, and 88.3% during the eccentric contraction, or when lowering a weight. For practical purposes, an average of about 89% overall.

The study also revealed that during the lifting, or concentric part of the exercise, the maximum intramuscular tension only lasted for between 0.25 and 0.5 seconds. For practical purposes, this is an average of about 1/3rd of a second during each isotonic repetition. This is because traditional isotonic resistance exercises naturally involve movement. They also have aspects of velocity and acceleration to consider in the overall equation. "Force" is only produced for a split second to produce a maximal contraction of the muscle fibres. The same research also showed that the level of muscle activation during isometric exercise was as high as 95.2% and that it lasted for the entire 7 to 10 seconds of each exercise. This is a huge increase over the 1/3rd of a second muscular activation achieved during a single repetition of weight training.

Therefore, based on these discoveries, technically, a single isometric exercise performed at only two-thirds of an individual's maximum can deliver similar or often even better results than the equivalent of up to 3 sets of 10 weight training repetitions in the lifting phase of the exercise.

To explain this further, I will use a typical barbell curl exercise in the lifting phase as my example, where the object of the exercise is to engage as many muscle fibres as possible in a maximum muscular contraction. Naturally, 3 sets of 10 repetitions give us an overall total of 30 repetitions. One set of 10 repetitions of the barbell curl in perfect high-intensity style produces a maximum muscular engagement for approximately 3.3 seconds. Three sets of 10 repetitions of the same exercise, a total of 30 repetitions, will give a total of approximately 9.9 seconds of maximum muscular engagement and an average of 89% muscle activation overall.

In comparison, one high-intensity isometric contraction exercise produces a maximum muscular engagement that lasts for the entire duration of the exercise. Even though the optimum time over which an isometric exercise is performed was found to be 7 seconds, this is almost always rounded up to the 10-second target number. The maximum muscular engagement will last for the entire 10 seconds of a high-intensity isometric exercise, with 95.2% muscle activation overall.

This is proof that is based entirely on scientific research that 3 sets of 10 near-perfect high-intensity curls when weight training, which takes several minutes to perform, still was not quite equal to the results achieved by a single 10-second high-intensity isometric curl exercise.

The Standard Isometric Contraction

The standard isometric contraction is a simple and highly effective technique. Therefore, we will focus on it for practical isometric training.

The standard isometric contraction, AKA: overcoming isometric contraction, AKA: maximum-effort isometrics, or whatever else you wish to call it, is when a muscle is applying force to push or pull against an immovable resistance. This is the most basic of all kinds of isometric exercise, and it is highly effective. This type of isometric contraction exercise was performed during the experiments by Dr T. Hettinger and Dr E. Muller at the Max

Planck Institute. It is also the technique referred to in their book The Physiology of Strength.

In a standard isometric contraction, it is theoretically possible to exert up to 100% of one's maximum capacity effort against an immovable object and then continue to hold that level of force throughout the exercise. This means that standard isometric contraction can be a very high-intensity exercise system.

Performing an isometric exercise against an immovable object at a certain level of force for a given duration of time will teach your body to recruit more muscle fibres to try to move the object. As you perform the exercise and generate as much force as possible, your CNS, or Central Nervous System, learns that it needs to activate and recruit more muscle fibres to reach the goal of moving the object.

Since this will naturally be impossible to move, the process will continue each time you exercise to make you stronger and grow more muscle. Your body mechanisms become trained to readily activate and recruit additional muscle fibres when facing similar challenges, which, in turn, repeats the cycle more readily every time.

As we mentioned earlier, the immovable/solid object can be anything completely solid and safe to use. This can be a wall, a door, a door jamb, a parked motor vehicle or anything similar. Perhaps the most common objects used to enhance everyday isometric exercise training are sturdy towels, climbing ropes, martial arts belts, scuba diving weight belts, webbing straps, golf clubs, and broom handles, etc. All the aforementioned items are excellent when used properly and will deliver some excellent results. More importantly, they are typically readily available for most people, which makes exercising with them so much easier.

Another common way to perform isometric exercise is to do it in a self-resisted way. Self-resisting means pushing or pulling against your limbs/hands/feet, etc. For example, you might place the palms of your hands together at chest level with your hands roughly at the midpoint of your body. In that position, you would then press your hands together using your chest muscles to provide the primary driving force, and then you would perform a highly effective self-resisted isometric chest press!

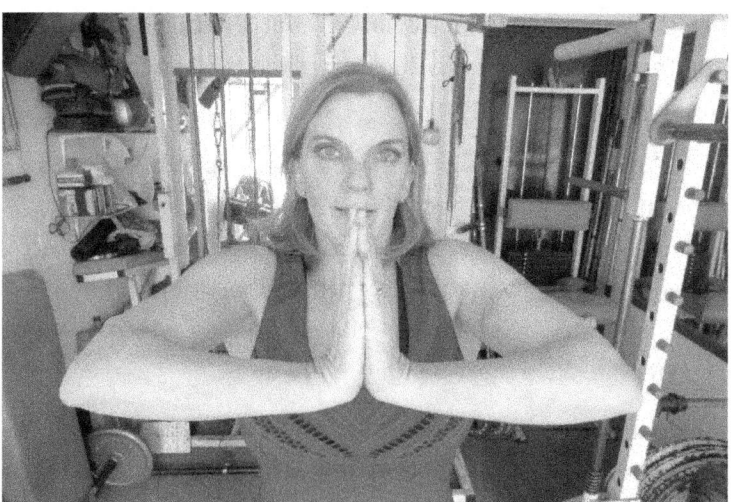

It is possible to perform a well-balanced and highly effective self-resisted isometric workout to exercise virtually every section of the body. So, never underestimate self-resistance exercise because it can be immensely powerful indeed. Also, self-resistance exercises are an excellent way to ensure that a personal maximum resistance is used safely and with minimum risk of injury caused by applying too much force.

The fact is that it does not matter which method is chosen. It can be isometrics performed against an immovable object, self-resisted isometrics, or a combination of the two. The most important thing is that either the object must be completely immovable through human muscle power alone, or the force of one body part must be able to completely counterbalance the force of another body part to produce a muscular stalemate.

Intensity, Force, Strength, and Power

Intensity will always be a relative term, and it is often completely misunderstood when used regarding exercise. When it comes to exercising your muscles, intensity is the percentage of your ability to move a resistance. Technically, an individual's highest possible level of intensity is when they reach a point of momentary failure after exerting themselves completely.

However, the important questions we need to try to answer are: "How hard is hard?" and "How intense is intense?" To some degree, both are very subjective. Taking two people of roughly equal fitness, something that is intense to one person might be considered comparatively easy to the other.

Hard is a relative term, and handling 50 lbs of resistance is impossibly hard if your strength is only at the level required to lift 49 lbs. However, if you can lift 100 lbs as a maximum, then lifting 50 lbs is going to be comparatively easy.

Often, the only factors differentiating between people and the intensity level exerted are mental toughness, determination, and perception.

Therefore, to gain the greatest benefits from isometric exercise, the first thing that must be learned is how to determine, with a reasonable degree of accuracy, what level of intensity is being applied to an exercise.

It is just a fact that what one person deems to be 100% of their capacity will always be quite different from another person's estimate. The accurate estimation of what one person deems to be 2/3rds of their overall maximum intensity will also vary from person to person. The accuracy of estimation will also vary greatly between an experienced professional athlete and an absolute beginner to exercise.

Experience has taught us that most people who are new to exercise will always fall well short of accurately estimating any given percentage. A beginner will find it more challenging to accurately estimate what 2/3rds of their 100% maximum is compared to a more experienced athlete. Many people might believe they are performing at 100% capacity when they are only performing at around 2/3rds, or perhaps at only 50% or less of their 100% maximum.

This is because exercise is new to them, and therefore, the experiences and feelings in their bodies associated with it are also new. They simply have no common frame of reference when it comes to calculating/estimating their level of physical exertion.

31

The human brain has a built-in mechanism that helps to protect the body and prevent it from performing a physical activity to such a level that it could cause serious damage or even death. This is the mechanism that makes your brain tell you to stop exercising when it begins to get tough, and the feeling of wanting to stop exercising only increases as you continue to push yourself harder to do more. This is all despite the biological fact that you are physically capable of doing much more than is being suggested by the messages you are receiving from yourself.

Over time, the brains of people who exercise regularly, especially at high intensity, will naturally adjust and reposition this built-in safety margin. This means that the brain of an experienced high-level athlete does not "tell" them to stop an exercise until the level of intensity is much higher than it would be for a beginner.

Therefore, how is it possible to subjectively quantify and then impart appropriate levels of recommended intensity when it comes to exercise? This problem is even more challenging when one considers that accurately translating and subjectively assessing various intensity levels will always be subjective to every individual.

If you were to train as hard as humanly possible, with near 100% maximum intensity, which involves super-strict form and training to complete failure and beyond, then you simply could not train for a long time. It is just physiologically impossible. Physics and biology are quite simple in this respect.

The intensity of your workout is directly proportional to the length of time you can physically perform it. The harder and more intensely you exercise, the shorter the time you can physically perform it.

Make no mistake, performing a 7-second isometric exercise while exerting close to your personal 100% maximum physical capacity is completely and utterly exhausting, even for a professional athlete.

What does all this mean when it comes to accurately communicating various levels of exercise intensity, especially when there is no professional coach or elaborate and expensive measuring equipment at hand?

Research clearly shows that almost everyone will stop exercising long before they are in any danger of becoming seriously fatigued. Most people will *think* they are exercising at a much higher intensity than they would if they were only a little more mentally resilient.

This does not mean that people should suddenly begin pushing themselves beyond their physical limits, which would be stupid. However, it does mean that most people who enjoy a higher-than-average level of mental resilience, determination, and being in physically good condition can push themselves much harder than they might think. If anyone ever feels "genuine" strain or fatigue to the point of becoming injured, then they should stop exercising immediately.

Even without the aid of a professional coach to monitor, encourage you, and measure your intensity and progress with specialist equipment, the tips we have outlined in this section will help you get the most out of every workout. It is also worth remembering that if you cheat, then the only person who loses is you.

As a footnote, for the sake of clarification, exercise intensity refers to how much energy is expended when exercising, including the amount of weight used per repetition. Perceived intensity varies with each person. Intensity and force are technically different, but are frequently accepted as interchangeable terms in the common vernacular.

Muscular strength is different from muscular endurance, which is the ability to produce and sustain muscle force over a certain period of time. While strength is the maximum force you can apply against a load, power is proportional to the speed at which you can explosively apply it. In other words, it is the ability to quickly produce a given amount of force.

Muscular force, often referred to as muscular strength, is the physical power exerted by muscles to perform various actions, such as lifting, pushing, or pulling objects. It results from the contraction of muscles and is vital for human mobility and functionality.

Technically, How Does a Muscle Grow?

How does a muscle grow? This is one of the most common questions concerning fitness and exercise. However, it is also one of the most misunderstood concepts, even amongst fitness professionals and personal trainers. To see for yourself just how uninformed or badly informed some people are, simply join one or two of the social media groups online so you can read some of the absolute drivel posted by 'keyboard warriors' who purport to be 'experts' on the subject. Alarmingly, many of these people seem to have developed a hardcore following, which to the science-based professional is like watching 'fools leading other fools' on a wild goose chase.

So, back to the key question, which is, how does a muscle grow? To explain this, we must examine three concepts: 1) muscle growth through increases in the volume/size of myofibrils inside the muscles, commonly called myofibrillar hypertrophy. 2) hyperplasia, which is when there is an increase in the number of muscle cells/fibres. 3) Sarcoplasmic growth, which is all about increasing the fluid content.

When it comes to exercise, the muscles you wish to grow must be challenged with a workload greater than they can currently accommodate. In other words, an exercise that is intense enough to stimulate growth. This stimulus can come from any source, such as lifting a heavy object, weight training, isometrics, compressing a spring in a device such as a Bullworker™, or through self-resistance, either hand-to-hand or limb-to-limb or using an Iso-Bow™, etc.

This process creates trauma to the muscle fibres, disrupting the muscle cell organelles. This then triggers other cells outside the muscle fibres to greatly increase in numbers at and around the point of the trauma to repair the damage. The process of repair involves a fusion of cells. This, in turn, causes the cross-sectional area of the muscle fibre to increase because the muscle cell myofibrils increase in both size and quantity. This process is more commonly known as hypertrophy. Since this process increases the number of cellular nuclei, the muscle fibres generate more myosin and actin. These are contractile protein myofilaments, which help make the muscle stronger.

This is the basis of what is more commonly known as myofibril muscle growth. In addition to this, there is also probably a process called hyperplasia. I use the term 'probably' because this concept is extremely controversial for many reasons. One of the key problems is that evidence of this in human beings is lacking, whereas there is a mass of evidence supporting hyperplasia in mice and other animals.

Hypertrophy is the increase in the size of the existing muscle fibres to accommodate the increased demands placed upon them through intense exercise. Hyperplasia, concerning skeletal muscle growth, is the increase in the number of muscle fibres, which in turn will also increase the cross-sectional area of a muscle.

Despite a lack of evidence supporting hyperplasia in human beings, logic supports the process. This is because of a theory known as Nuclear Domain Theory. This states that the nucleus of a cell (a muscle cell in this instance) is only able to control a finite area of cellular space. It is thought that satellite cells donate their nuclei to the muscle cell until a certain point is reached when this can no longer take place.

Beyond a certain limit, and through continued intense training, the cell must eventually divide to create two cells instead of the former single cell. When this happens, the entire hypertrophy process starts over once again. This probably means that most of the muscle growth is almost certainly caused by hypertrophy, and a much smaller percentage can be attributed to hyperplasia at any given point in the muscle stimulus/growth process.

Finally, the subject of sarcoplasmic muscle growth needs to be addressed. Sarcoplasmic muscle growth is the increase in the volume of sarcoplasmic fluid in the muscle cell. These fluids and energy resources surround the myofibrils in your muscles, containing mostly glycogen together with other elements, including creatine, ATP, and water.

To clarify, glycogen is simply a type of sugar that serves as a form of energy. It is deposited in bodily tissues as a store of carbohydrates, and it is the body's main form of storage for the sugar glucose. Glycogen is stored in two main places in the body, one being the liver and the other being the muscles.

More importantly, glycogen is the body's secondary source of long-term energy storage, with fat being the primary energy storage source. When glycogen is in the muscles, it is converted into glucose for use as energy when performing sports, etc., and glycogen stored in the liver is converted into glucose for use as energy throughout the body and in the central nervous system.

Therefore, sarcoplasmic growth increases muscle volume, but this increase is not in functional strength mass since it does not increase the number of muscle fibres. It is like 'the pump' in that it increases the size and shape of the muscle through the muscle holding an increased amount of fluid.

Rest Time Between Exercises

Naturally, the rest time between exercises during a workout is quite different from the rest and recovery needed to allow your body to respond positively to the stimulus generated by exercise.

If you keep the rest time between exercises brief enough, the workout routine itself will give you an excellent cardiovascular workout, and this is what we recommend that you ultimately aim for. If you are already very fit, we recommend that instead of performing the optional cardio routine, you simply put more effort, force, and intensity into each isometric exercise.

At the same time, aim to keep the rest time between those exercises as brief as possible. This approach will help you work towards performing each exercise with an Ultra-High Intensity Ultra-Short Burst™ effect, which will greatly improve your overall fitness level and boost your Base Metabolic Rate (BMR).

However, if you are not already fit, you may wish to begin by simply allowing each isometric exercise to deliver all the cardio you need as you gradually build up your fitness and endurance levels. This gradual approach ensures that you feel confident and reassured in your fitness journey. Eventually, you will increase your fitness level to a point where you can gradually reduce the rest time between each exercise to a minimum that works best for you.

Once you have learned how to fully engage the muscles during each exercise with sufficient force, and at the same time, you have learned how to breathe fully, deeply, and naturally throughout each exercise. At the same time, you should be keeping the rest time between exercises to a minimum because this combination will have an excellent and beneficial cardiovascular effect.

Dynamic Flexation™

Dynamic Flexation™ is a technique we devised to help ensure that we gain maximum benefit from the isometric portion of our exercise regimens. I will recap and briefly summarise the Dynamic Flexation™ technique as originally laid out in "The 70 Second Difference™" book.

We always recommend that everyone who performs any kind of resistance exercise practice some form of Dynamic Flexation™ before performing any exercise. This will help ensure that all muscles, tendons, ligaments, joints, and spine have become naturally and properly engaged in the correct biomechanical exercise position.

We would never recommend that you immediately apply maximum power and force as soon as you assume any exercise position. This is unless you are a very experienced athlete or unless you are training with a qualified coach to perform a certain type of isometric exercise to develop extra power, such as a static-dynamic or explosive/ballistic isometric technique. Instead, we recommend that you always breathe naturally as you gradually flex and engage your muscles and joints into performing the exercise.

To perform Dynamic Flexation™, you gradually flex your grip and the muscles you are about to exercise while applying an increasing level of force immediately before performing the exercise. The exercise is then performed, and to disengage from it, we recommend reversing the Dynamic Flexation™ engagement process.

We prefer to gradually apply tension and force to the exercise through Dynamic Flexation™, typically for between 2 and 3 seconds, or even for as long as 4 seconds if needed. This all takes place before beginning to count the required 7-second exercise time of the isometric contraction.

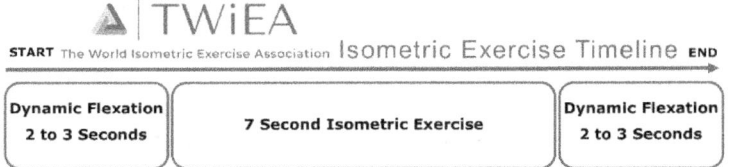

We prefer using one deep, full breath in and out to count each second that has elapsed more accurately. This way, you will time each exercise more accurately and not be tempted to hold your breath at any point, which is a mistake that beginners often make.

Similarly, at the end of an exercise, we do not recommend that it be ended abruptly. Instead, we recommend reversing the Dynamic Flexation™ technique so that you gradually relax as you slightly move each muscle and joint out of the exercise position.

This process helps enormously because when you are in a good position, you will gain the maximum benefit from each exercise you perform.

Dynamic Flexation™ is when you move and adjust your feet, legs, hips, and especially your hands as you gradually assume a solid position and handgrip. As you flex and move, you will be making micro-adjustments.

All exercises will be performed best if you assume a correct and solid handgrip, fist clench, or foot position, etc. One of the most important aspects of assuming the correct exercise position begins with your grip.

Without a solid grip on a bar, handle, or anything else you need to hold while exercising, you will naturally be setting yourself up to perform sub-maximally. You can also help develop injuries, which can include sore elbows, joints, ligaments, and tendons.

Dynamic Flexation™ is a concept that embraces the broader principles of motor unit recruitment and "Henneman's Size Principle" to increase the contractile strength of a muscle.

Elwood Henneman's principle stated that under load, the motor units in a muscle are engaged according to their magnitude of force output, from the smallest to the largest, and in task-appropriate order.

This means that the slow-twitch, low-force, fatigue-resistant muscle fibres are activated before any fast-twitch, high-force muscle fibres are engaged, which are less fatigue-resistant. Since the body naturally works in this way, it enables precise and finely controlled force to be delivered at all output levels.

This also means that fatigue will always be minimised when exercising or performing tasks in daily life. It will also be proportional to the sequential engagement of the most appropriate muscle fibres.

41

Isometric Exercises and Blood Pressure

Some exercise critics point out that performing an isometric exercise raises blood pressure. However, these people conveniently forget that the same is true of all other forms of exercise, including freehand callisthenics and traditional isotonic resistance training with weights.

ALL physical activity, especially exercise, will cause your blood pressure to rise for a short time. Providing that you are in good health, if you always breathe deeply, naturally and normally when performing any exercise, any rise in blood pressure will soon return to normal when the exercise stops. The faster this happens, the fitter you are.

For advanced athletes and/or those who have been used to hard and intense isometric training for a long time, you will already have made significant progress in strengthening your heart and circulatory system.

For those who are new to isometric training, just like with any form of exercise, the best way to get into it is by taking it slowly and less intensely at first. Newcomers to exercise, especially isometrics, should always focus on applying less force and breathing fully and deeply throughout all exercises. NEVER HOLD YOUR BREATH!

Under strict medical supervision, even those with Coronary Artery Disease and high blood pressure should be able to increase their physical activity levels with a reasonable degree of safety. However, if you already suffer from high blood pressure, you should always exercise at a much lower level of intensity than someone who has no physical issues.

FURTHERMORE, EVERYONE, ESPECIALLY PEOPLE WITH HYPERTENSION OR ANY FORM OF CARDIOVASCULAR DISEASE, SHOULD ALWAYS CHECK WITH THEIR DOCTOR BEFORE BEGINNING ANY KIND OF EXERCISE ROUTINE.

Rest and Recovery

Many factors must be considered when calculating your ideal recovery period. These include your age, current health and fitness level, the quantity of exercise you have done, and, most importantly, the intensity of the exercise.

Some people need a recovery period of between 24 and 48 hours; for others, it may be as brief as 12 to 24 hours. As a rule, the recovery period will always incrementally increase as the intensity of the exercises increases towards an individual's 100% potential maximum capacity. Always be aware of this, and make sure that you factor this into your rest and recovery time calculations. The diagram will help to outline this.

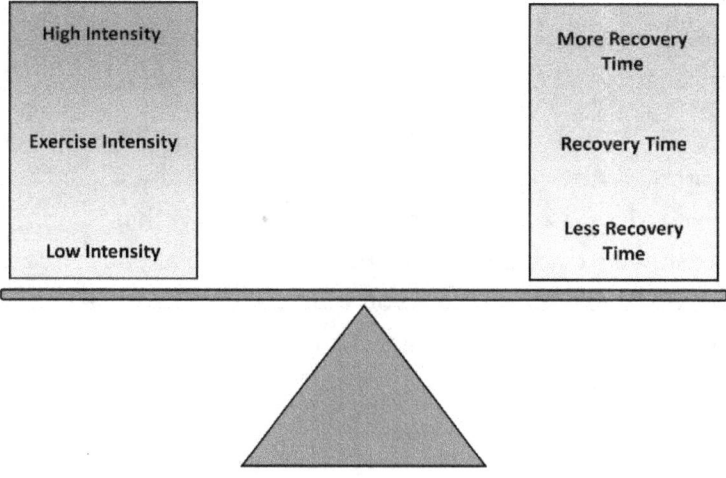

Sports scientist J. Atha's research revealed something remarkable. It showed that the average person could safely perform an exercise like this daily without overtraining when performing isometric contraction exercises at two-thirds of an individual's maximum capacity. Standard isometric contraction exercises can be safely performed daily by almost anyone of almost any age and in almost any physical condition as a means of strength development, body shaping, and even bodybuilding.

However, we recommend a full rest day between sessions for more intense workouts due to the higher demands placed upon the central nervous system (CNS) and the time needed to recover and fully benefit from the exercise. Several other factors affect post-exercise recovery. These include a balanced and properly executed stretching routine and getting enough quality sleep. While you sleep, your body releases certain hormones that help you repair and rebuild damaged tissue and will directly help your muscles grow.

Adequate Nutrition is Vital

Quality post-exercise nutrition will help your body repair itself faster, decrease your recovery time, and maximise the benefits gained from the exercise. Research shows that post-exercise immunodepression peaks if you exercise longer than you are currently capable, and problems are enhanced due to reduced or inadequate nutrition.

Hydration is also one of the most important factors in recovery and overall health, especially since muscles are mostly composed of water.

Early studies suggested a 30 to 60-minute window after exercise when you need to eat, after which your body begins to draw upon itself to repair and recover from your workout. Later studies found that this window can be anything from 1 to 3 hours, depending on the workout type, applied force, overall intensity, and goals. On average, since most leave 60 minutes after food before hard exercise, and if a workout lasts an average of 45 minutes, then a 30 to 45-minute window to eat after exercise will mean it has been up to 150 minutes (2.5 hours) since your last food; therefore, the earlier suggested 30–45-minute window still makes sense for most people especially if they want to build more muscle and strength.

Most people mistakenly consume excessive amounts of protein at the expense of other key nutrients, such as carbohydrates. Therefore, in doing this, they are working against their best interests and overall optimum health. One of the key nutrients that has been found to help enormously when in recovery from prolonged periods of heavy exercise is carbohydrates. A lot of research supports the hypothesis that carbohydrate is the most important nutritional factor in preventing post-exercise immunodepression. Most do not realise that the protein composition of human muscle is typically only somewhere in the region of between 18/9% and 21% protein (average 20%), and the rest is made up of water, glucose, lipids, and carbohydrates, etc. We will not go into more detail here; however, if you want to learn more about this and many other surprising nuggets of useful information about sensible nutrition and exercise, then they can be found in The 70 Second Difference book.

Strength, Stamina, Endurance, and Resilience

Understanding the difference between strength, stamina, and endurance is important because once you do, you will be able to devise the most suitable workout routines for your body type.

Muscular strength is possibly best understood as a muscle's capacity to exert force against resistance or weight. This is comparatively easy to measure because one's ability to lift a given amount of weight for a single repetition is a good measure of strength.

Stamina is the length of time at which a muscle or group of muscles can perform at or near their maximum capacity. For example, the number of squats you can perform with a given weight that is 90% of your maximum would be a measure of your stamina or the distance that you can carry a similarly heavy object, such as an anvil.

Endurance is all about time and your ability to perform a certain muscular action for a prolonged period, regardless of the intensity at which you are working.

Resilience is all about your ability to recover from whatever stresses and demands are placed on your muscles. However, resilience is mostly all about your state of mind, your mental toughness and ability to endure, perform and deliver under pressure, and how you recover quickly emotionally.

Your body's muscular composition will always determine your performance in certain sports. The amount of slow-twitch muscle fibres you possess will determine your performance at endurance-related events, and both type A and type B fast-twitch muscle fibres are all about explosive power and your ability to maintain it.

In simple terms, if you possess mostly slow-twitch muscle fibres, you will naturally be better suited to endurance sports. Alternatively, you are a natural weightlifter if you possess mostly fast-twitch muscle fibres.

It is important to note that no matter what your natural predisposition might be in this respect, with the correct training regimen, it is still possible to significantly increase your abilities in your naturally weaker opposing areas of speciality.

Biceps, Supination, and Strong Arms

When most people think about the biceps muscles, they only think about flexing the biceps and elbow joints to create a classic bodybuilder pose. However, there is a great deal more to the biceps muscles than this. While flexing the arm in the way I have just described might be a primary function, another equally primary function is the action of twisting the forearm and hand, otherwise known as supination. This is it in pictures.

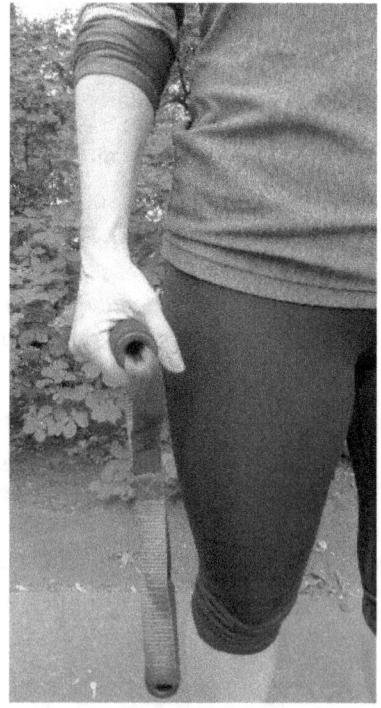

Neutral Position Front

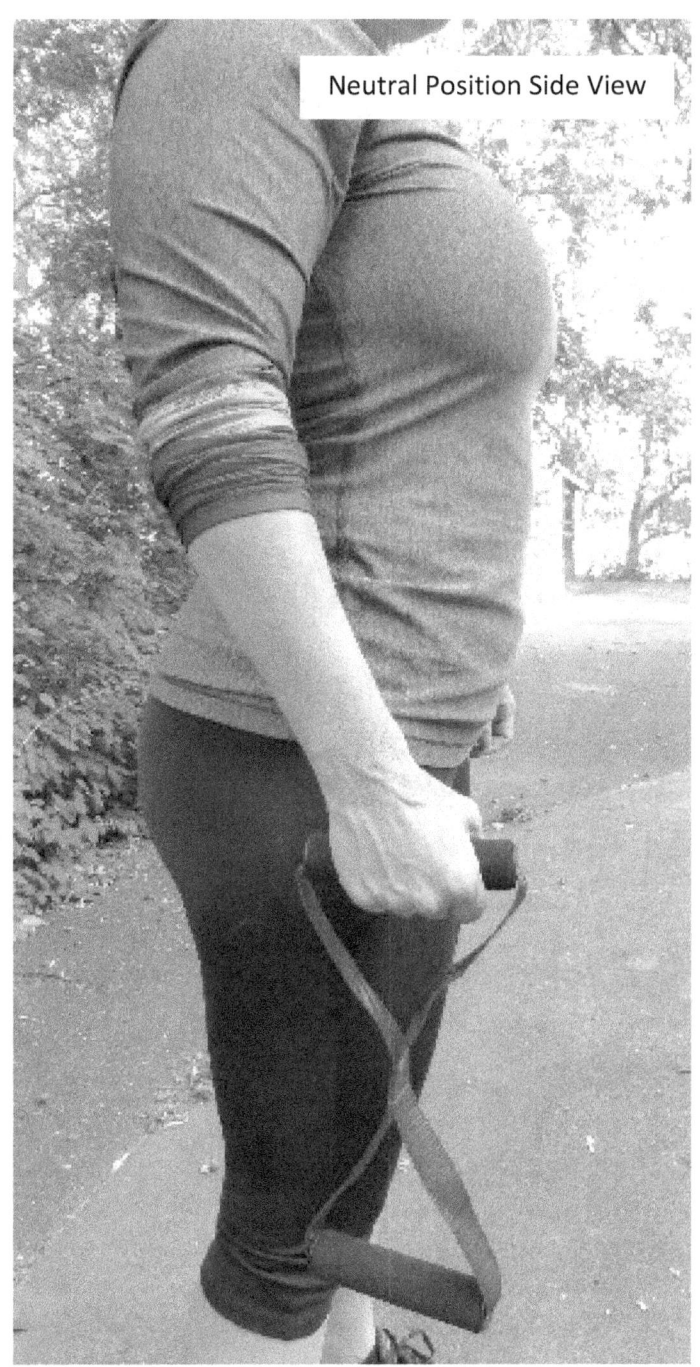

Neutral Position Side View

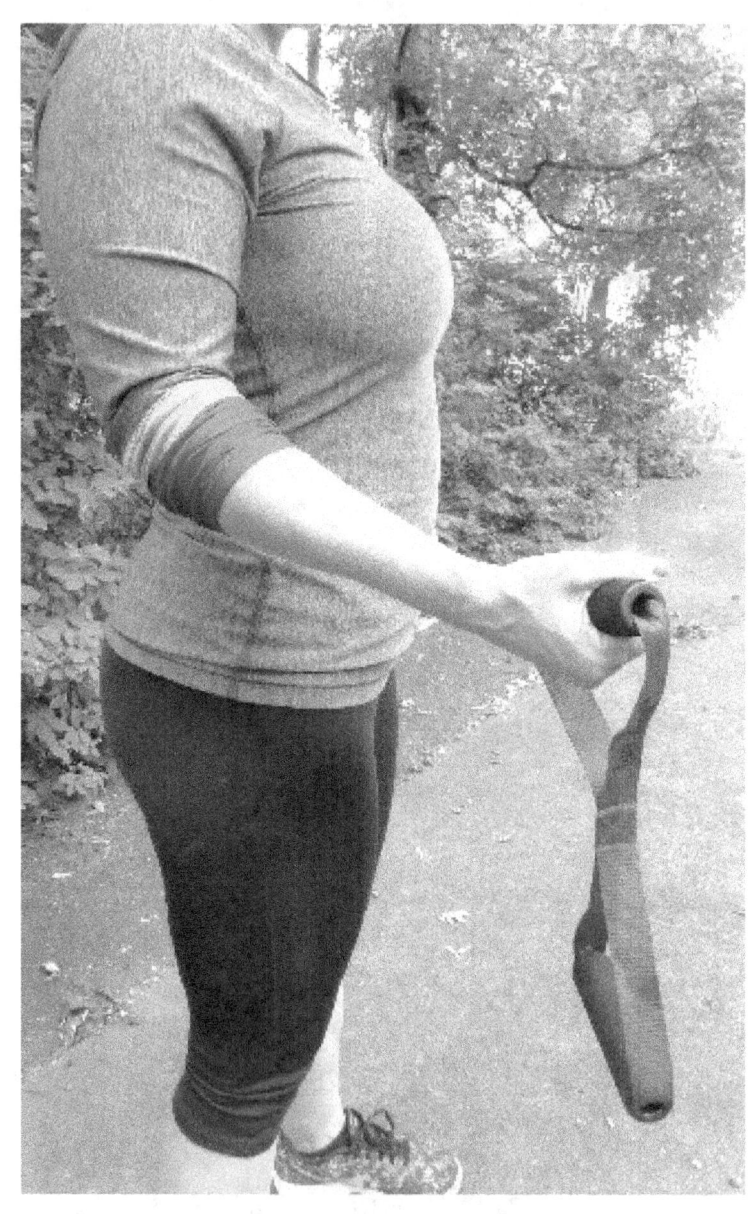

Mid Supination Side View

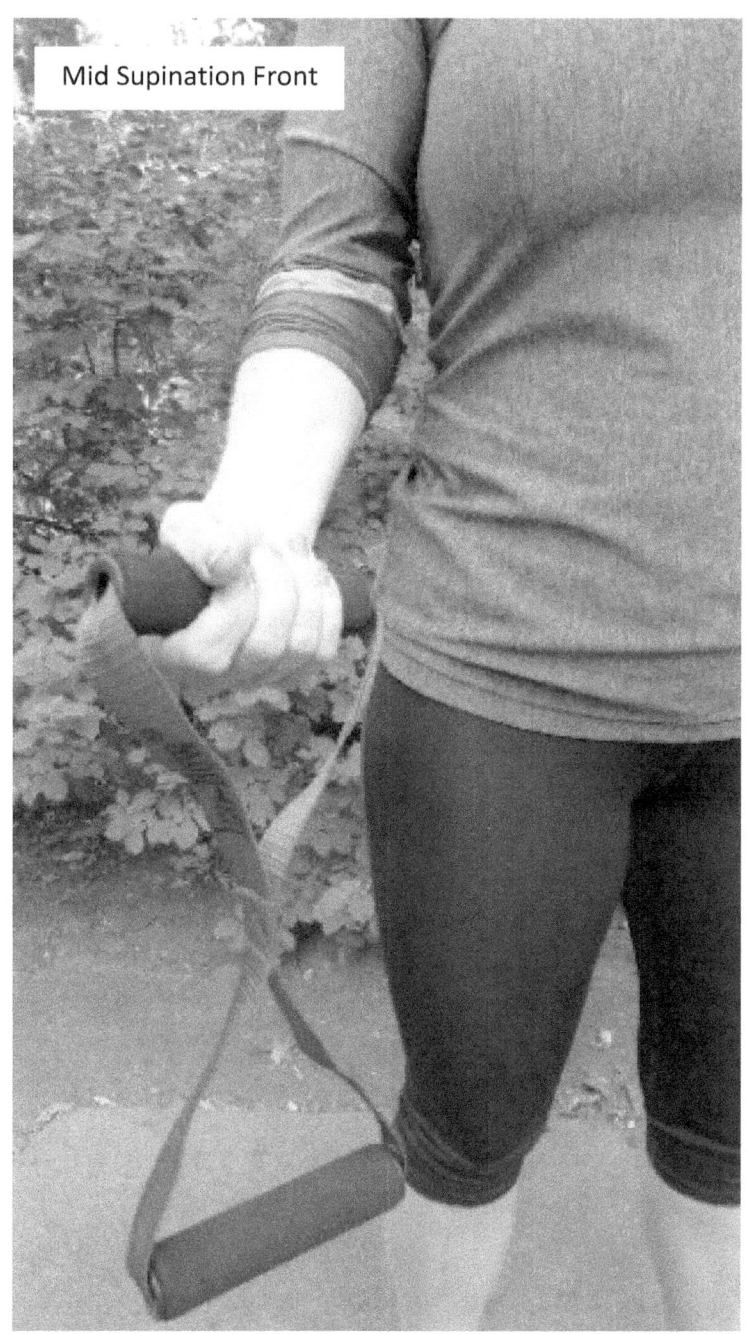

Mid Supination Front

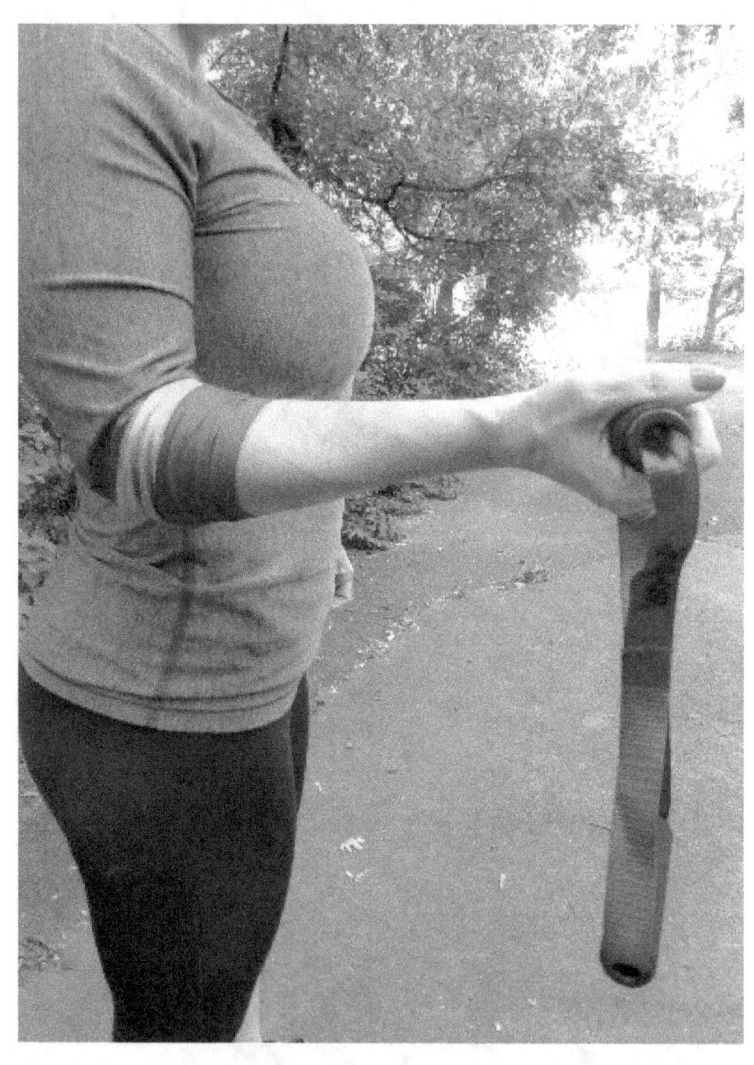

Full Supination Side

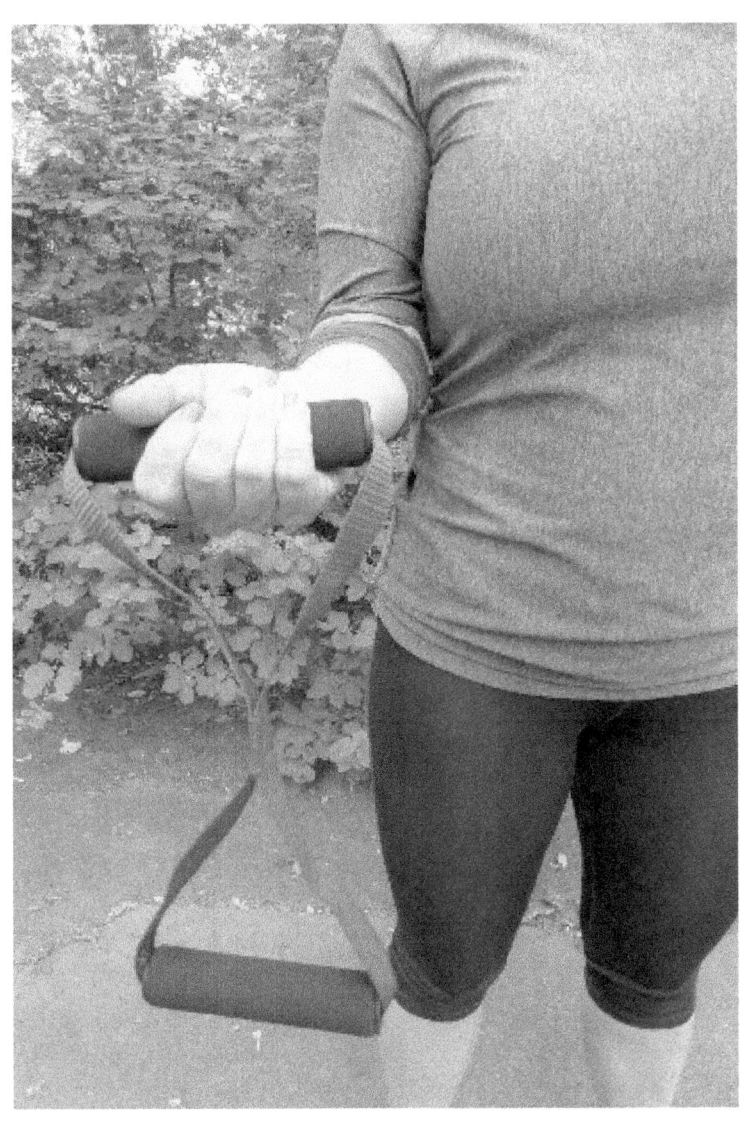

Full Supination Front View

Supination starts with the hand in a neutral position, roughly parallel to the side of your upper thigh. You twist it as you raise it until your palm is facing upwards at the top of the movement when the biceps are fully flexed. As most people think, the brachialis muscle is the primary mover of elbow flexion, not the biceps brachii.

This is because, even though the biceps brachii "show" muscle is seen flexed during a classic biceps pose, the brachialis that underlies it generates about 50% more power than the biceps brachii. Therefore, supination is important not only for elbow rotation but also for overall upper arm strength.

Therefore, you must consider all component muscles and their actions to gain maximum benefit and strength when exercising your overall front upper arm. The problem with isometric exercise in this respect, when pitting one limb against another limb or against a static, immovable object such as a wall, door or chair, is that it does not naturally allow the brachialis muscle to be exercised effectively. This is where the iso-Bow® fills the gap and enables a range of exercises to be performed in a neutral, partial, or fully supinated position.

- ▲ As a general rule, never allow your elbows to move forward or kick out to the side when performing a biceps curl.
- ▲ As with all curling exercises, never allow your wrist to bend backwards to fall out of alignment with the forearm because, in this position, you are between 3 and 4 times weaker than if your hand and wrist were locked in the correct biomechanical alignment.

53

Chapter 4: Helen's Transformation

In 2014, I found myself suddenly single again. After a rocky 2nd marriage to an unfaithful husband, my self-esteem was at its lowest. I always thought I was a strong and independent woman, but with the thought of a 2nd divorce and losing my family, I had never even considered leaving him. That all changed in the blink of an eye.

My husband had suddenly moved back to his country, and within the next few months, I had to send my stepdaughter back to be with him. My two oldest kids, at this point, were now grown and following their dreams. I was completely alone; I did not know what to do with myself. As you might imagine, this was not exactly a "fun-filled" time in my life, and somehow, I felt like I had once again failed both my family and myself.

During those 10 months, my body weight "ballooned" to the heaviest it had ever been. The only saving grace was that, being in the fashion industry, I was always able to dress well and cleverly hide the excess weight I was carrying.

At first glance, to the untrained eye, no one could tell just how unfit I was; however, I felt it. I had a hard time climbing stairs and walking long distances, and I completely lacked both energy and enthusiasm, which meant that I just wanted to sleep all the time.

By this time, my twin sister, Rhonda, had also gained weight to the point where she had become 50+ lbs overweight, so she made a life change. She hired a coach and announced to the family that she would be entering a bodybuilding competition to compete in the Figure Class.

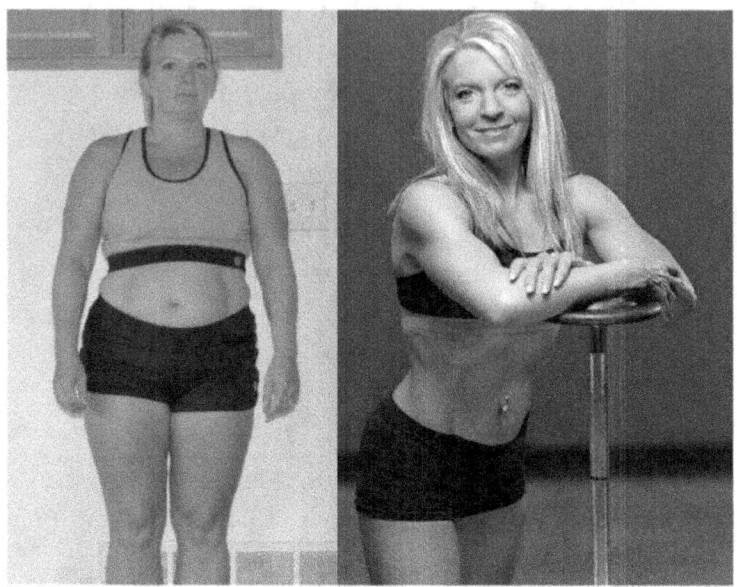

I was extremely proud of her for wanting to lose weight and build muscle. However, I also hate to admit that I was completely sceptical about her ever achieving her target weight and competing on stage in a bikini.

After about 10 months of training with weights and following a strict diet, I was completely shocked to find that she had done the unthinkable and lost that much weight!

She looked incredible, and I could hardly believe my eyes. It was at that point that I realised something profound. I realised that anybody could get into shape IF they want it bad enough and are determined enough. You just must commit the time, effort, and research needed to succeed.

Because of her amazing transformation, I was inspired to enter my first Bodybuilding Competition in a Bikini Fitness Class.

My best friend Glenda Ama and I decided to compete together. We agreed that we were ultimately responsible for the size and shape of our bodies and made a pact to hold

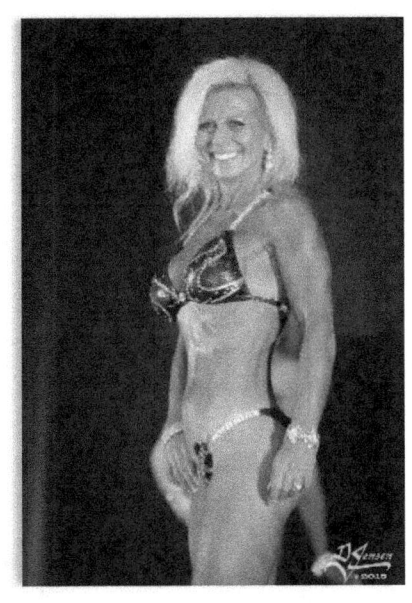

each other accountable if we strayed from the plan.

To compete, I needed to drop 40 lbs of excess fat, and she needed to drop 60 lbs, but my twin sister's

inspiration made us sure that we could do this! In only 8 months, we had done it! We had made our target bodyweight and our target body fat percentages.

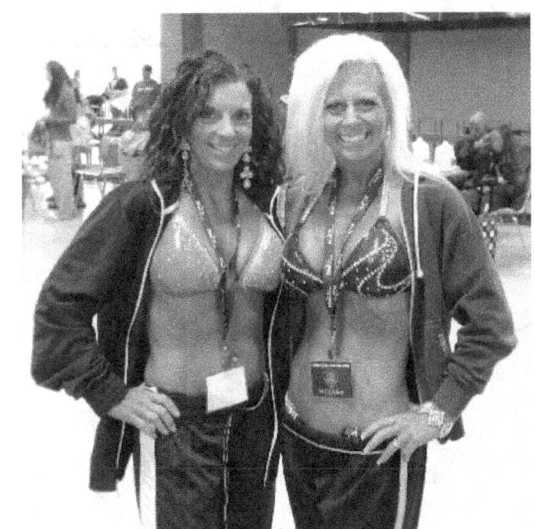

That year, we competed in our first of several competitions, and we both walked away with some trophies. I had achieved that which I thought once was impossible; I had dropped 40 lbs of excess fat, competed on stage in a bikini, and in the process, it earned me 2nd, 3rd and 4th place positions in the competitions I entered that year.

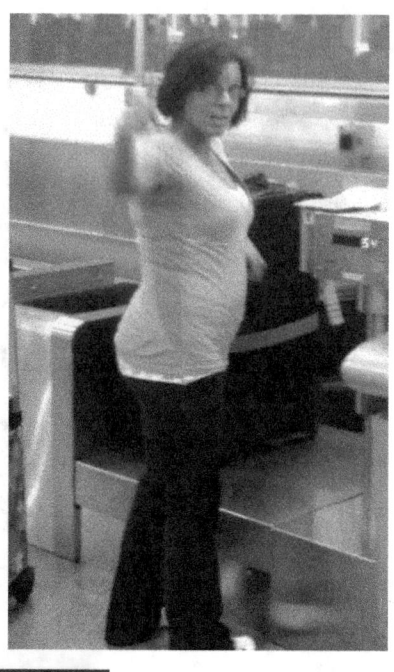

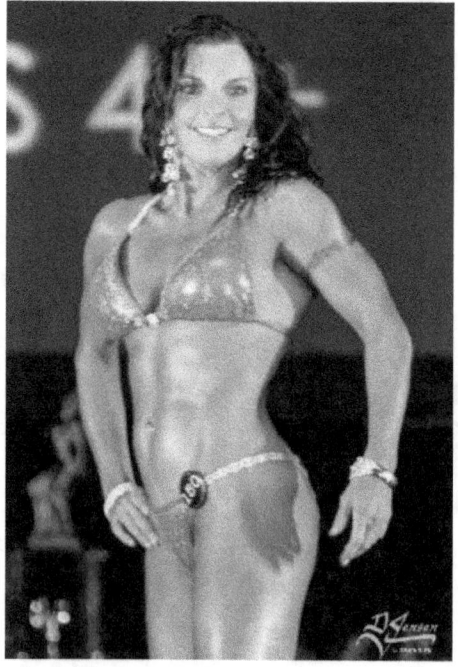

I had literally transformed myself in every way, and to do it, I only needed to keep an open mind and do a little research. If I had done this sooner, I could have led a much healthier, fitter life in my twenties and thirties.

Chapter 5: Transformation Gallery

The following pictures are from before my "transformation". They were taken when I had already lost 10 lbs, and I would suggest to anyone starting a workout routine to take pictures before you start to help track your progress. I certainly wish I had done that myself.

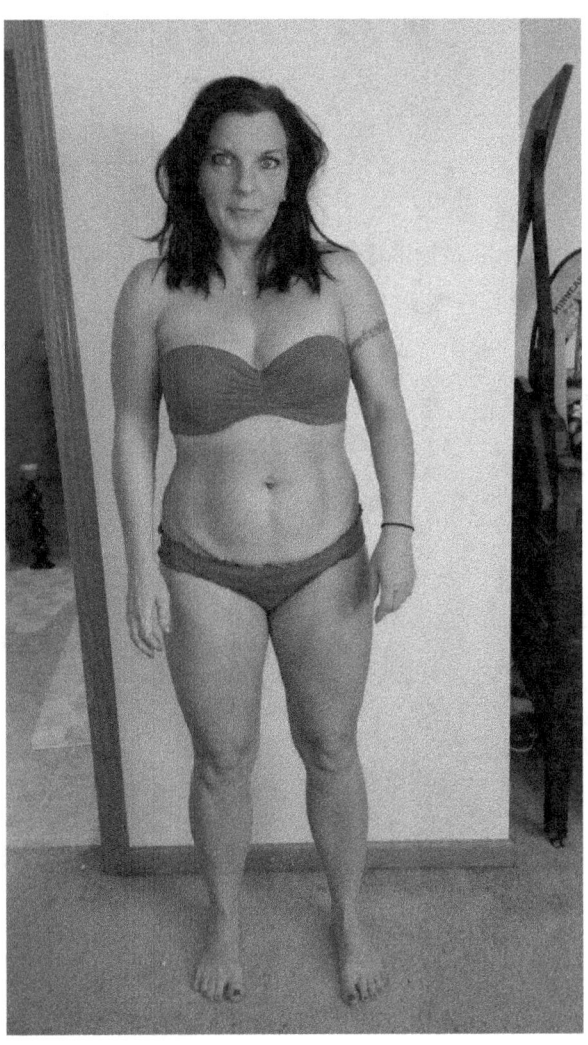

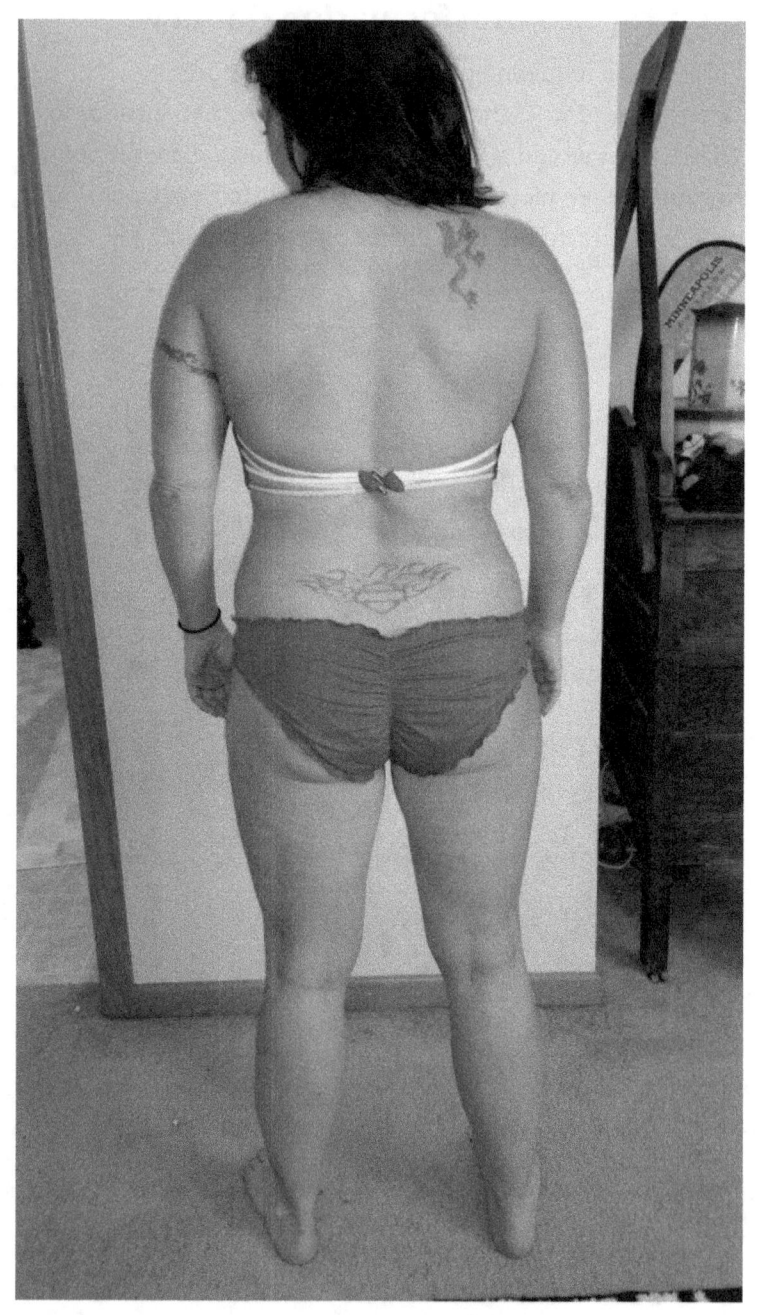

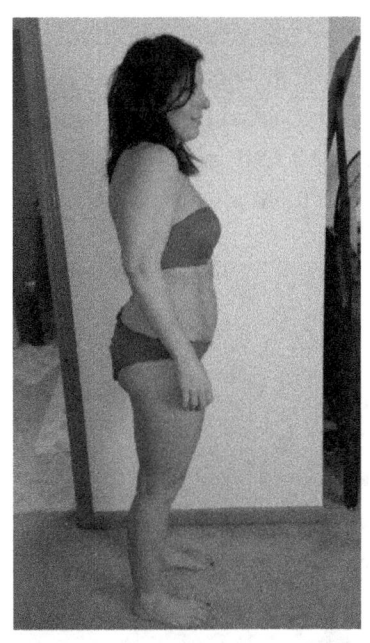
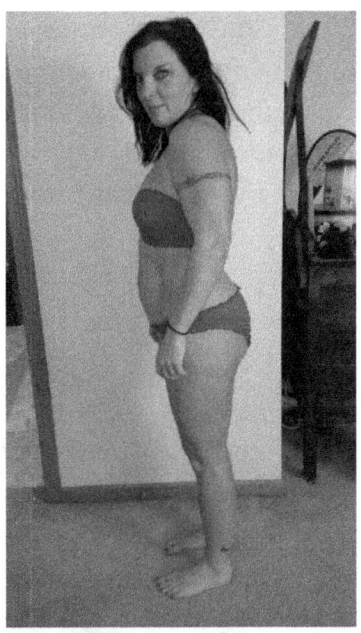
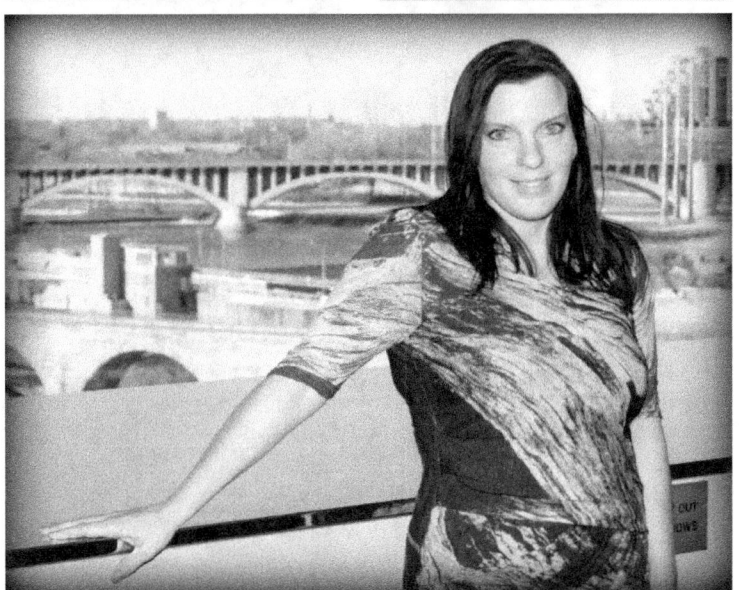

The results I achieved in my transformation photos required strict dedication to exercising six days a week and eating the right foods. When you decide to transform your body, you must fully commit yourself to it, which helps ensure that you get the results you have always wanted.

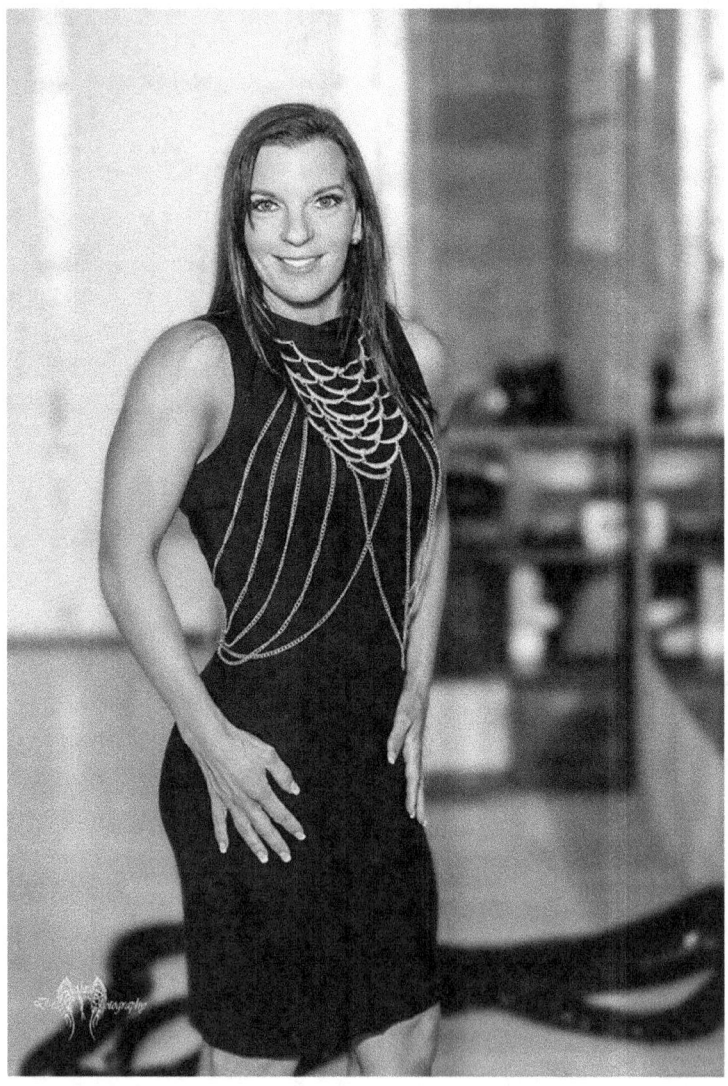

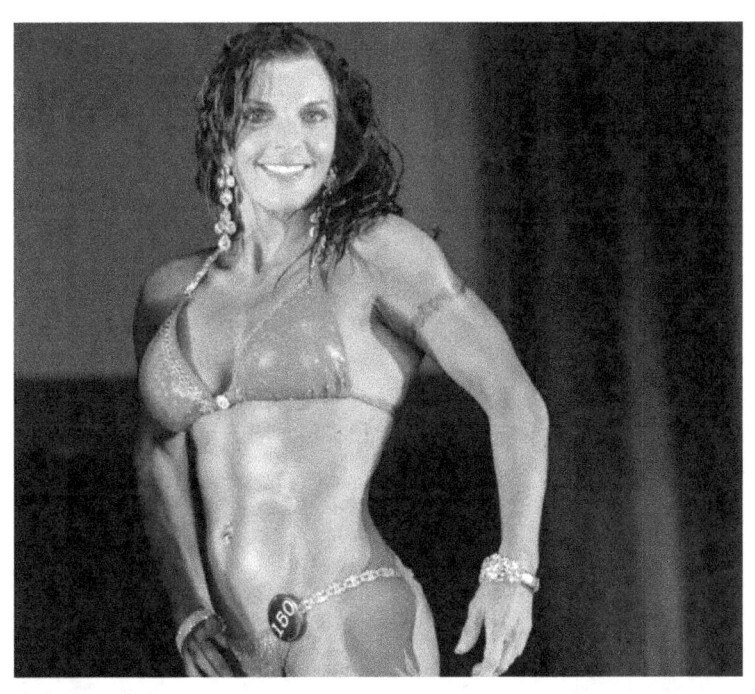

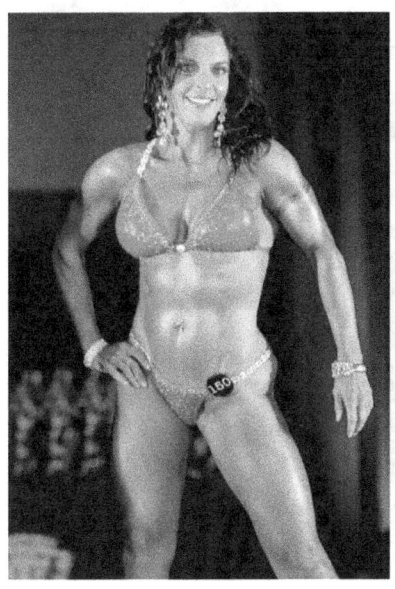

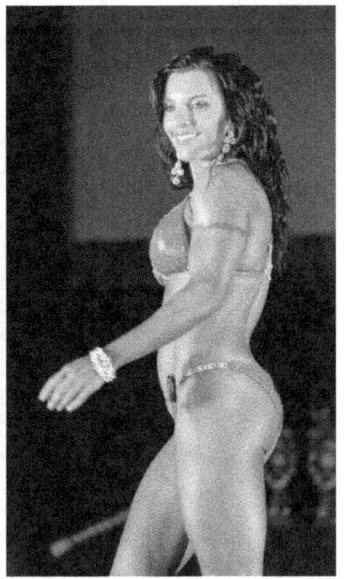

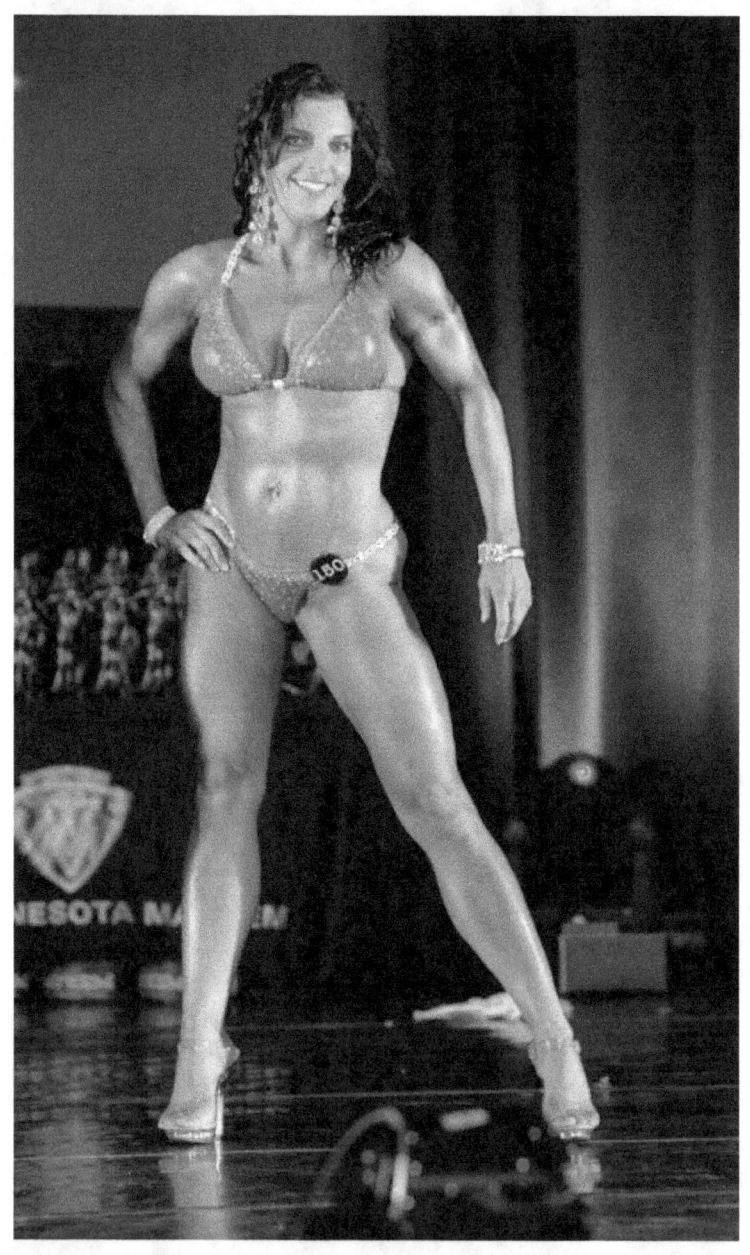

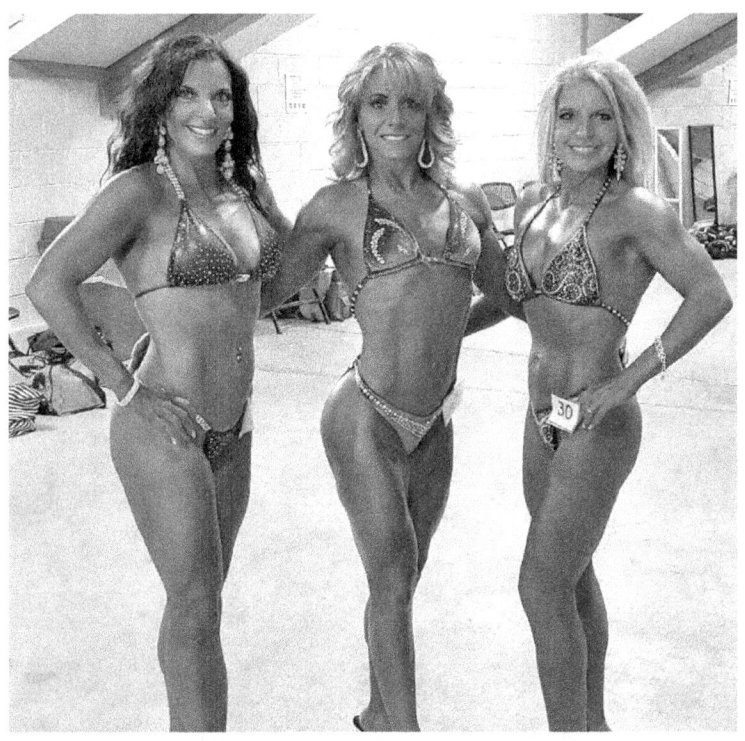

The photo above is special to me as I got to compete on the same stage as my High School best friend and twin sister! We are all 46 years old in this photo!

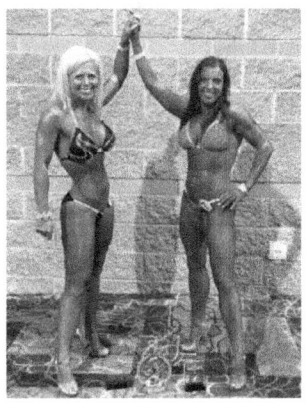

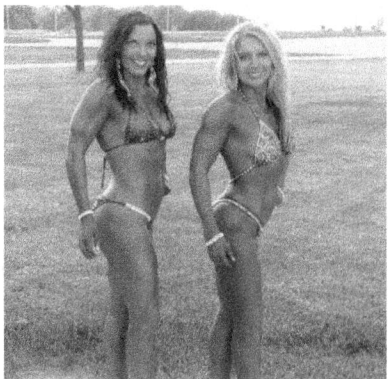

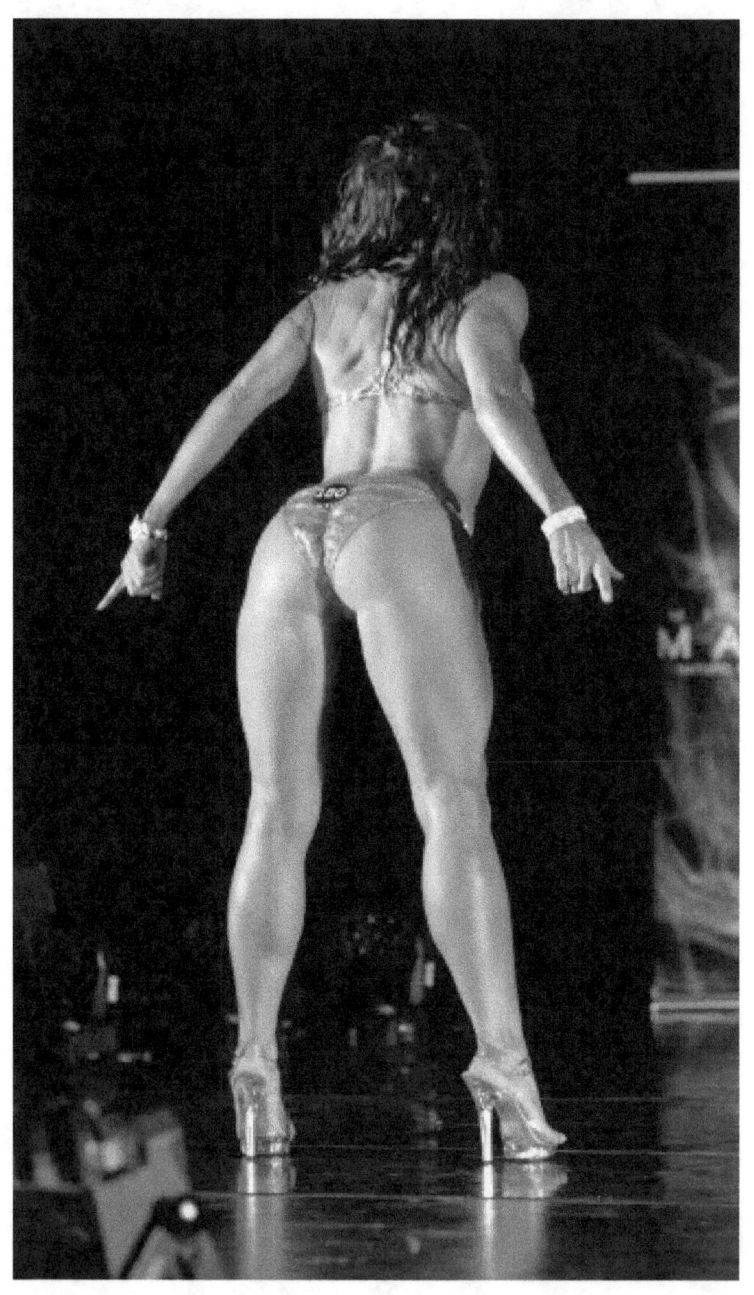

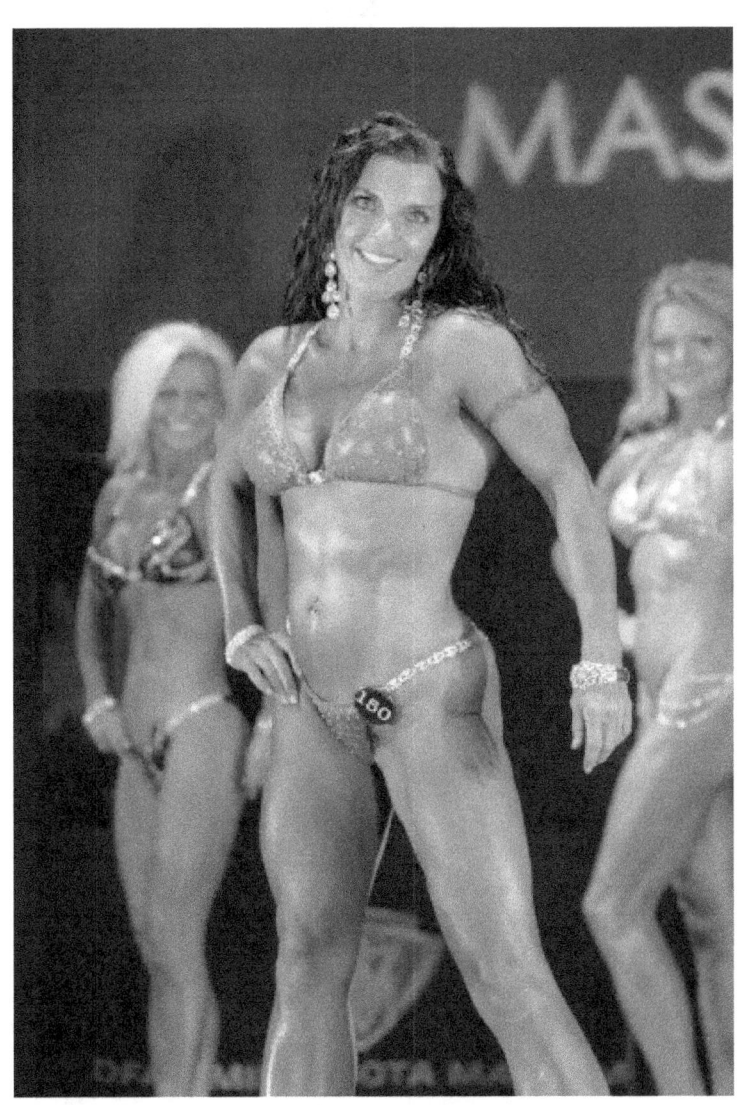

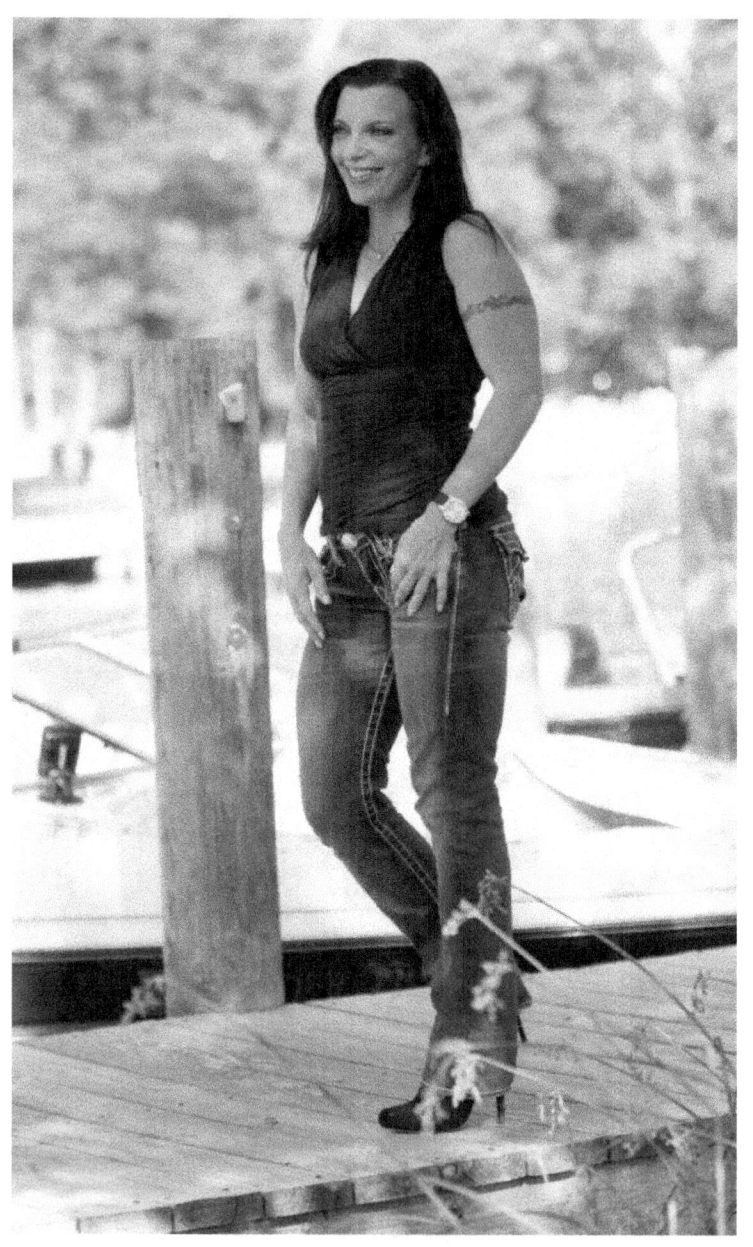

Chapter 6: All Things Iso-Bow®

We highly recommend and endorse the Iso-Bow®. as an exercise tool. This inexpensive little device is amazingly versatile and allows self-resisted isometric, isotonic, and functional isokinetic exercises to be performed easily. The Iso-Bow® provides the user with a biomechanically sound grip handle, which allows almost all exercises to be performed more effectively and with greater ease and comfort.

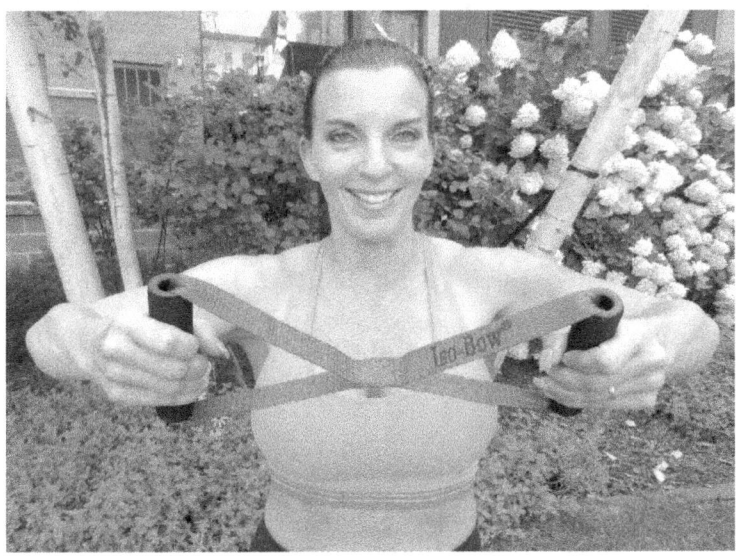

With a pair of Iso-Bows®, you can effectively exercise every major muscle group of the body and even perform advanced exercises such as pull-ups, the isometric squat, and the isometric deadlift. The level of workout you can get from using a pair of Iso-Bows® can range from an easy, low-level beginner's workout right up to a very high-intensity professional athlete level of workout. Amazingly, you can do all of this without any adjustment being needed to the Iso-Bows®. Each user will benefit proportionately, according to the amount of effort, force, and intensity that is applied during each exercise.

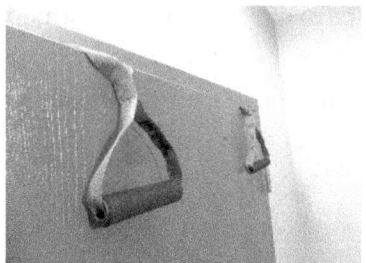 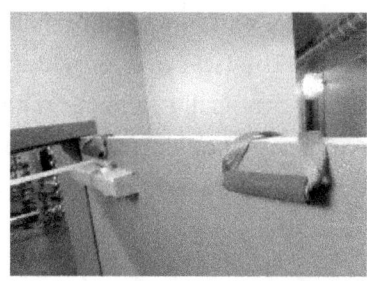

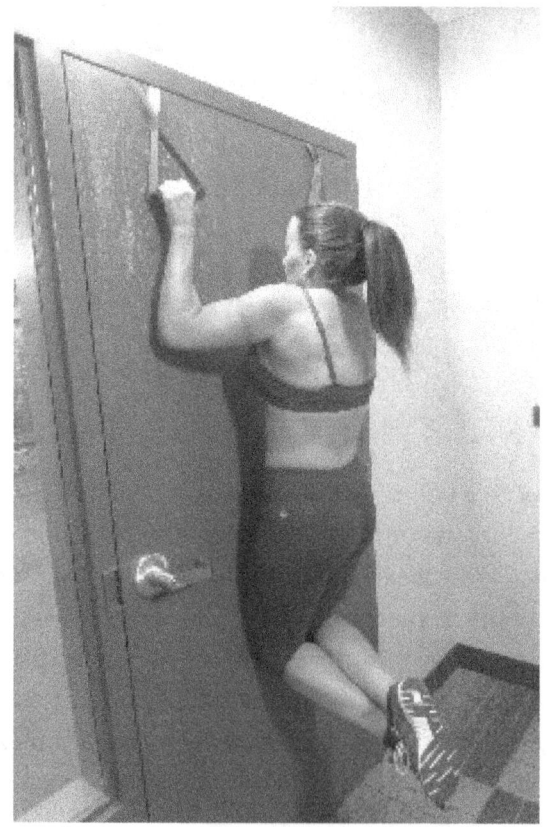

One of the standout features of the Iso-Bow® is its portability. It's so compact that it can easily fit into your pocket, handbag, briefcase, or backpack. This means you can take your workout with you wherever you go, making it the perfect companion for your busy lifestyle.

Perhaps the best-known of all isometric/isotonic home exercise devices is the Bullworker®, which has been a best-seller since its launch in the early 1960s. Today, it is still a best-selling device, and with good reason: It works. The smaller "partner" device is called the Steel Bow®, and both have interchangeable springs so that men and women of all strength levels and abilities can use them with roughly equal effectiveness.

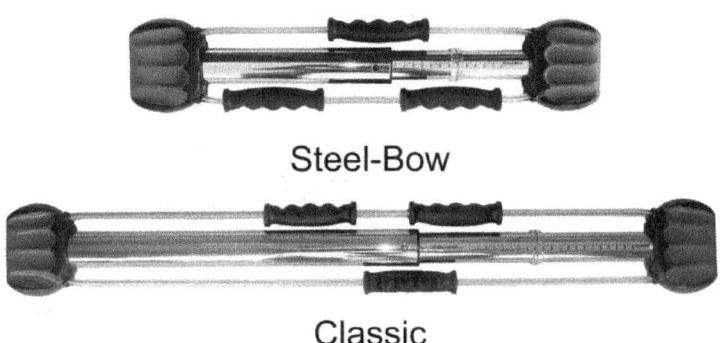

Steel-Bow

Classic

Securing the Iso-Bow® With Your Feet

When performing leg exercises such as squats and lunges, as well as lower back and glute exercises such as the deadlift, it becomes necessary to secure the Iso-Bow® using your feet properly.   There are several ways in which the Iso-Bow® can be secured using your feet, and your preference of how you do this will depend upon many factors, such as your foot size, choice of footwear, and ease of operation.

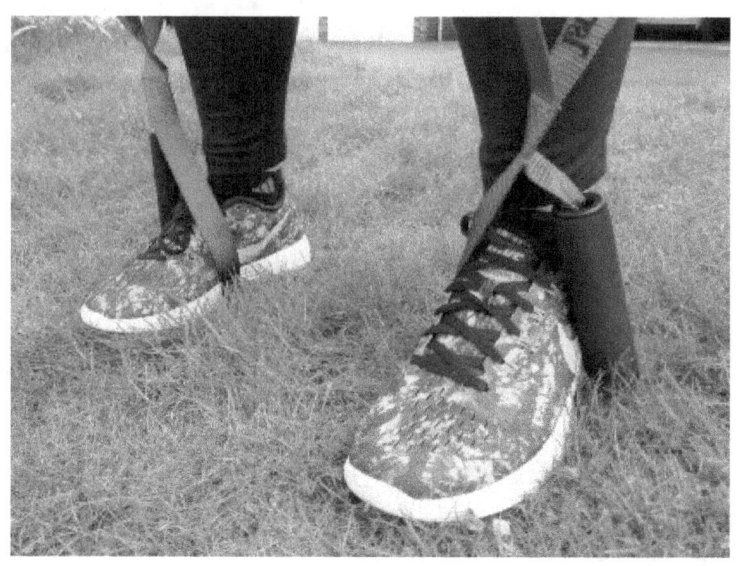

You can secure the Iso-Bow® with your foot inside one of the handles. To do this, adjust the handgrip to one side, usually the foot's outer side, and then place your feet inside the loop like a stirrup. Another method is to place the Iso-Bow® flat on the floor and then stand on one side of the straps so that the handle of the same side sits flush with your inner foot. In this position, your bodyweight combined with the handle pressing against the inner side of your foot enables you to pull safely and securely.

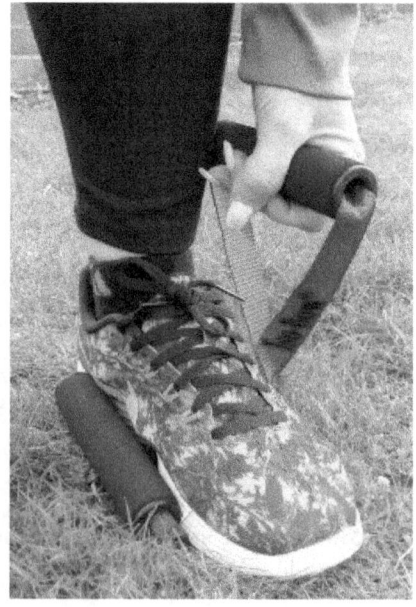

The final method is to simply place each foot through one end of an Iso-Bow®, stepping onto the foam hand grip as you do so. This method is slightly less stable than the other two methods. However, if the foot can be pushed far enough through the loop of the Iso-Bow® handle, then the handle will slightly raise the level of your heel, making it easier for some people to squat or lunge.

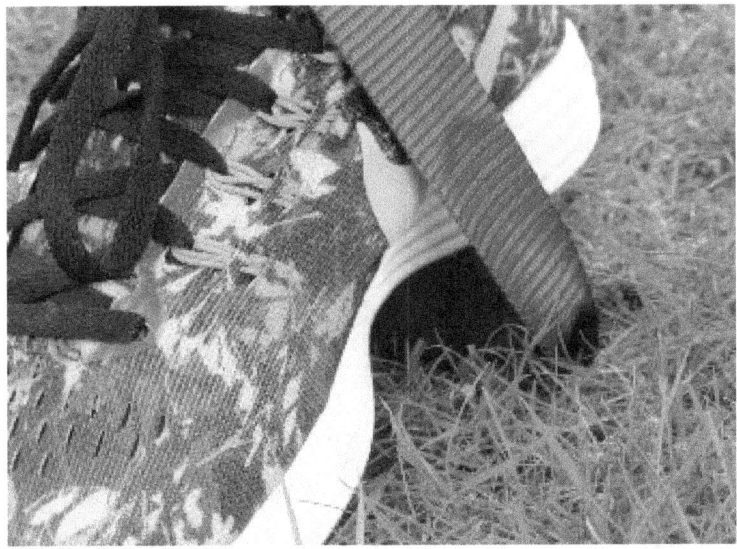

Naturally, safety is always a top priority, so whichever method you ultimately choose to use, always make sure that when securing the Iso-Bow® with your feet, there is never any chance of it slipping while you exercise.

Shortening The Iso-Bow® - The Cradle

Generally, the Iso-Bow® is the ideal size for most people to use with each exercise. However, occasionally, you may prefer to reduce its operational size by roughly half by creating what we call an Iso-Bow® cradle. To do this, place one of the handles inside the webbing loop of the other handle side of the device. The webbing then cradles the handle you have just placed inside the loop and can be gripped as normal. Your thumb and fingers can then wrap around the foam handle and the cradle loop's webbing to help create an even firmer grip position.

This reduced size allows for an even greater operational range within the movement capability of each limb/joint to be created for certain exercises. These include the Cross-Chest Press, the Upper Back Power Pull, and the Biceps and Triceps Cradle Press-Curl.

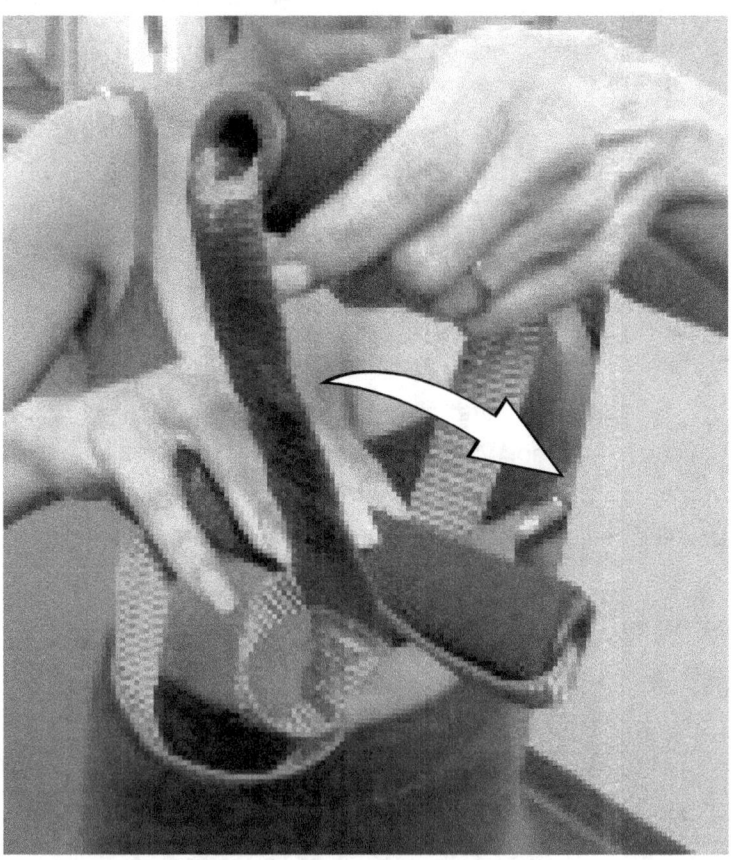

Charts of the Major Muscle Groups

The following charts showing the major muscle groups should help you to identify the ones you are targeting in each exercise more easily. The better acquainted you become with the muscle groups and their basic function, the better your exercise style should become.

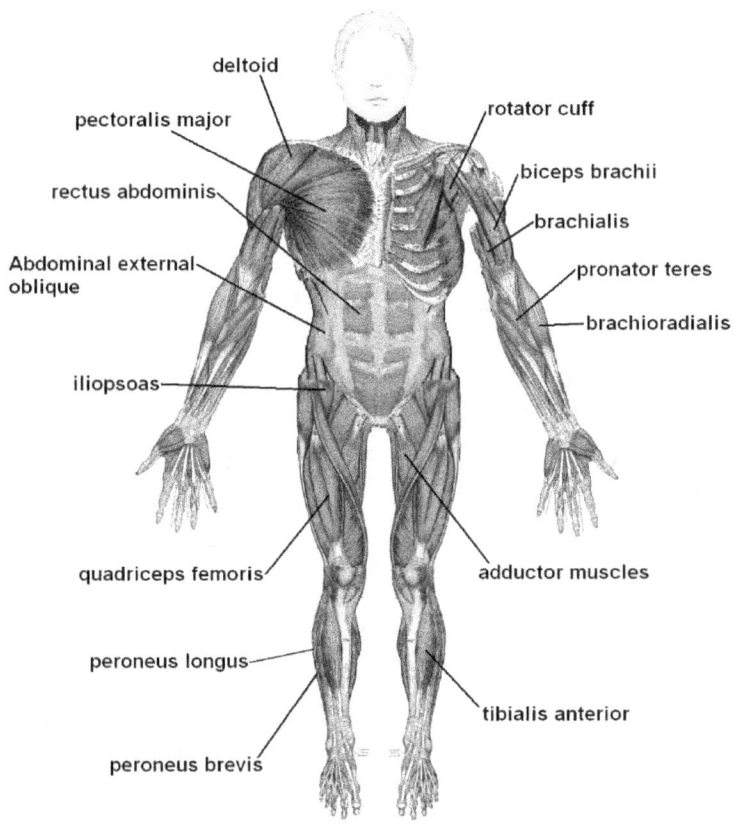

deltoid

pectoralis major

rectus abdominis

Abdominal external oblique

iliopsoas

quadriceps femoris

peroneus longus

peroneus brevis

rotator cuff

biceps brachii

brachialis

pronator teres

brachioradialis

adductor muscles

tibialis anterior

Frontal (anterior) View of the Main Human Skeletal Muscles

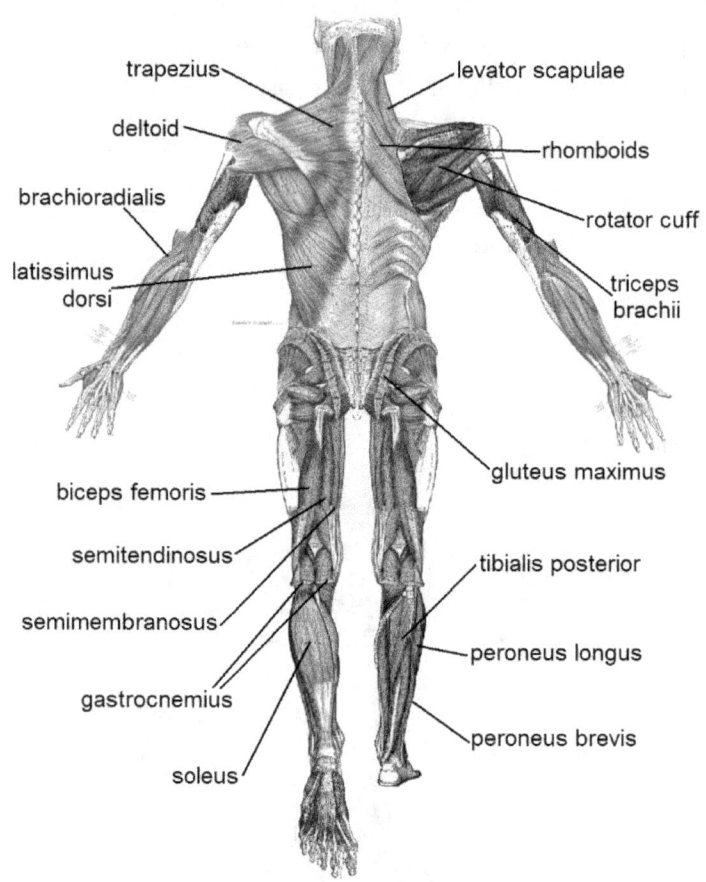

trapezius

levator scapulae

deltoid

rhomboids

brachioradialis

rotator cuff

latissimus dorsi

triceps brachii

biceps femoris

gluteus maximus

semitendinosus

tibialis posterior

semimembranosus

peroneus longus

gastrocnemius

peroneus brevis

soleus

Rear (posterior) View of the Main Human Skeletal Muscles

Chapter 7:

Things to Remember Before You Begin

- The first and perhaps the most important thing to remember is: **NEVER HOLD YOUR BREATH AT ANY TIME.**
- Breathing in and out naturally during all isometric exercises will also help you count the number of elapsed seconds much more accurately, with one full breath in and out taking approximately one second.
- We recommend that you read the instructions about each exercise carefully.
- Always leave a safe distance between you and others if exercising with any proprietary device or IIED (Improvised Isometric Exercise Device)
- Always check the structural integrity of any type of exercise device. If there is any doubt about the structural integrity, then do not use it for exercise or any other purpose.
- Before use, double-check that all adjustable joints on the exercise device and/or IIED are secure.
- Weight loss/fat loss will ONLY occur when any exercise plan is used in conjunction with a calorie-controlled diet.
- It is critically important to focus your mind on the exercise being performed completely. Envision the muscle you are exercising growing larger and stronger.
- Always consult a professional coach to devise a detailed stretching routine; this will ensure that you

are stretching the areas effectively rather than risking injury.

▲ Always ensure that a stable line of biomechanical progression is achieved before engaging in and performing any exercise.

▲ Warming-up, stretching, and cooling down are three of the most overlooked yet essential elements of exercise, and we cannot stress their importance strongly enough.

▲ During ANY form of physical exercise, including isometrics, if you apply too much force too soon, then you may inadvertently strain a muscle. Isometric exercise is particularly intense, and a single isometric exercise engages many more muscle fibres than even high-intensity weight training and at a much higher level.

For safety's sake, we always recommend using Dynamic Flexation™ to gradually and progressively engage your muscles in ANY exercise, especially isometrics, according to what we call The ISOfitness Exercise Engagement Timeline™.

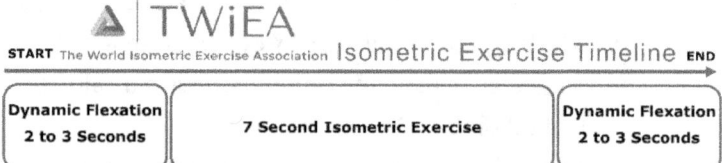

The main benefit of properly warming up for several minutes before a workout is injury prevention and increasing your heart rate and circulation to your muscles, ligaments, and tendons. It is important to remember that warming-up and stretching are two different concepts and that stretching is not a good warm-up. This is because stretching will put the muscle in an uncontracted position and weaken it. Stretching is always best performed after a workout has been completed, together with a proper cool-down. In addition to properly warming-up, always perform a gentle flex and stretch of the muscles and joints that are about to be exercised. For example, squatting down fully to flex the thighs and loosen the knees is always a good idea before performing any leg exercises. Dynamic Flexation™ performed before any exercise should help to ensure greater flexibility and increased blood supply to the muscles and surrounding tissue.

Isometric exercises are deceptively powerful. Even when engaging in what may feel like only moderate-intensity exercise, you are probably still engaging and contracting many more muscle fibres than you would in a similar isotonic exercise. If you have any doubts, always perform the exercise with less force. All exercises and workout plans work equally well for men and women, and both can build strength, muscle, body build, or simply get into great shape, each according to their natural ability.

In our exercise resource books, the exercises listed are suggestions of what can be performed for each body part/muscle group. We do not suggest that they all be performed. Instead, users may wish to select the most suitable exercises from each section. In our course books, please perform the exercises according to the workout session notes. **Finally, please reread and review the 'Important General Safety and Health Guidelines' section to ensure that you have fully complied with all recommendations. Only start using the isometric or any exercise system with the full approval of your physician.**

Chapter 8:
BEGINNER SSASS™ WORKOUT

Perform only one 7-second isometric exercise contraction.

⚠ Before you begin the full isometric contraction part of the exercise, take between 2 and 3 additional seconds to perform Dynamic Flexation™ to help you properly engage the muscles and joints. Similarly, at the end of each isometric exercise, do the same in reverse as you disengage from the exercise over between 2 and 3 seconds.

⚠ Perform the workout every day, taking weekends off or every other day, alternating with the 70 Second Difference Workout.

⚠ Take two days of rest over the weekend before starting the workout routine again on the following Monday.

BASIC SQUAT

To perform the basic Iso-Bow® supported squat, stand with your feet shoulder-width apart.

Bend your knees as far as you are comfortably able to, bending only from the hips and keeping your back straight.

Hold both handles of an Iso-Bow® and place the centre comfortably over the top of the thighs, close to the knees, to support some of your body weight.

Breathe naturally and deeply in and out for about 10 full breaths, which will take about 1 second per breath. Aim to perform an exercise breathing count of no less than 7 seconds and no longer than 10 seconds.

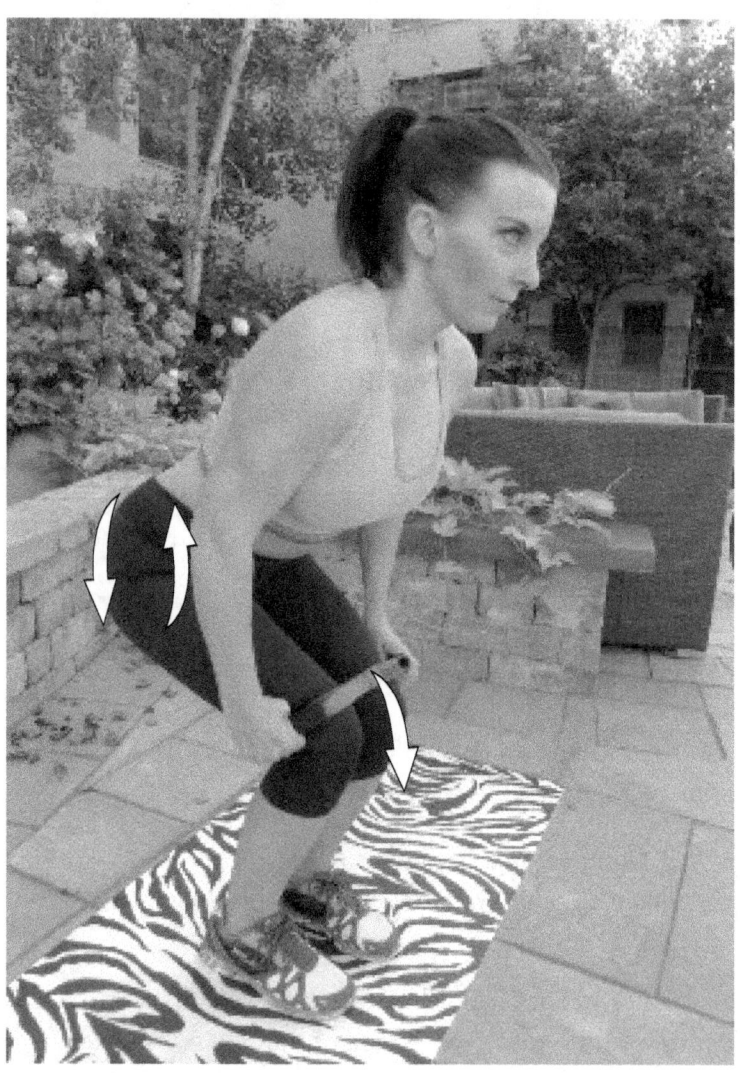

BASIC DEADLIFT

Stand with your feet shoulder-width apart and with your knees slightly bent. Bend forwards only from the hips as low as you are comfortably able to and hold both handles of

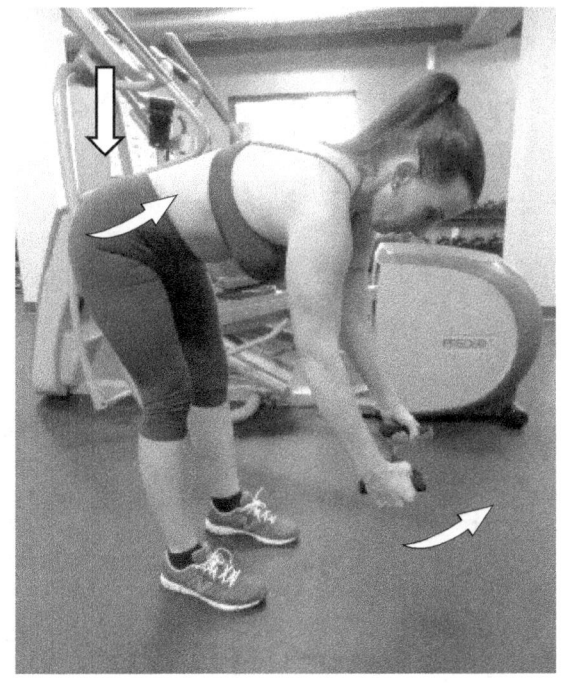

an Iso-Bow® downwards towards the floor.

Breathe naturally and deeply in and out for about 10 full breaths, which will take about 1 second per breath. Aim to perform an exercise breathing count of no less than 7 seconds and no longer than 10 seconds.

Only raise your arms if you are comfortable. In the same position, extend your arms and hold the Iso-Bow® straight out in front of you as far as you are comfortable to aid your balance and increase the resistance on your lower back muscles.

Breathe naturally and deeply in and out for about 10 full breaths, which will take about 1 second per breath.

Aim to perform an exercise breathing count of no less than 7 seconds and no longer than 10 seconds. Repeat the exercise with the other leg.

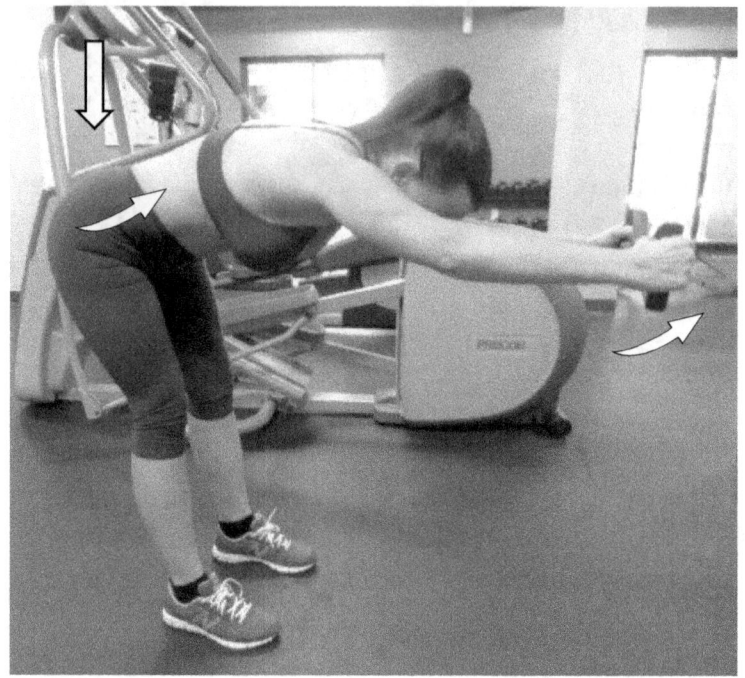

BASIC SIDE LEG LUNGE – LEFT AND RIGHT LEG

Bend one knee out to one side at about a 90-degree angle to create a side leg-lunge position.

Hold an Iso-Bow® and place it comfortably across the thigh of the bent leg, just above the knee, to help reduce the resistance on your thigh muscles.

Breathe naturally and deeply in and out for about 10 full breaths, which will take about 1 second per breath.

Aim to perform an exercise breathing count of no less than 7 seconds and no longer than 10 seconds. Repeat the exercise with the other leg.

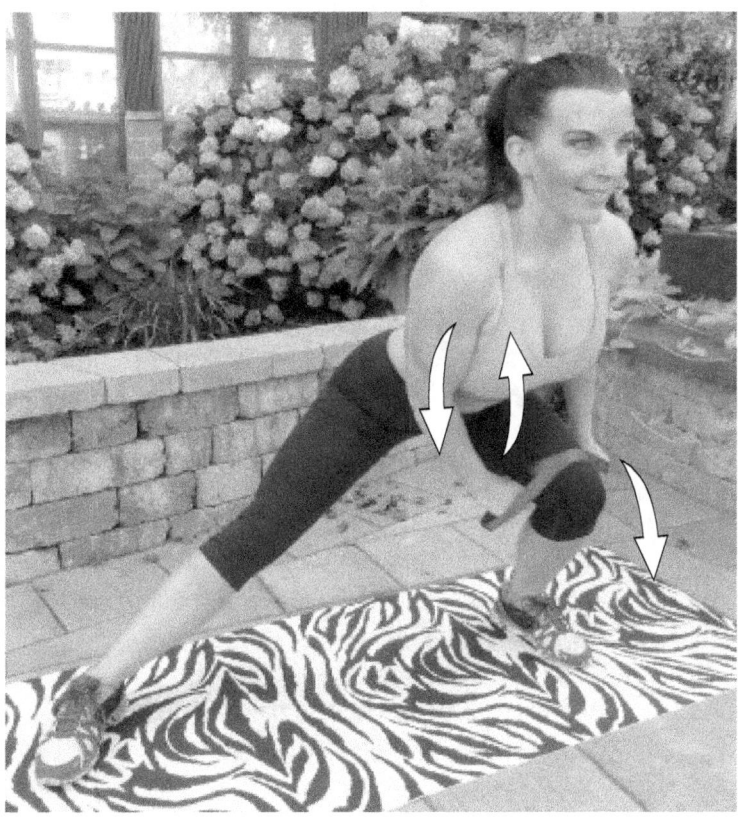

BASIC FORWARD LEG SPLIT SQUAT – LEFT AND RIGHT LEG

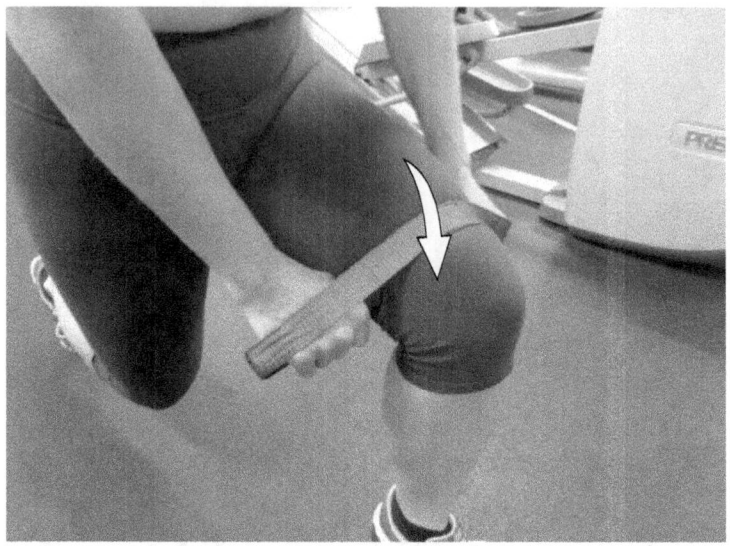

Stand with your feet shoulder-width apart to perform the basic forward split squat.

Bend one knee forward to about 90 degrees while moving the other leg backwards, with your trailing knee close to the floor, to create a split squat position.

Hold one Iso-Bow®, with the handles facing downward, and comfortably place it across the thigh of the extended leg, just above the knee, to help reduce the resistance on your thigh muscles.

Breathe naturally and deeply in and out for about 10 full breaths, which will take about 1 second per breath.

Aim to perform an exercise breathing count of no less than 7 seconds and no longer than 10 seconds. Repeat the exercise with the other leg.

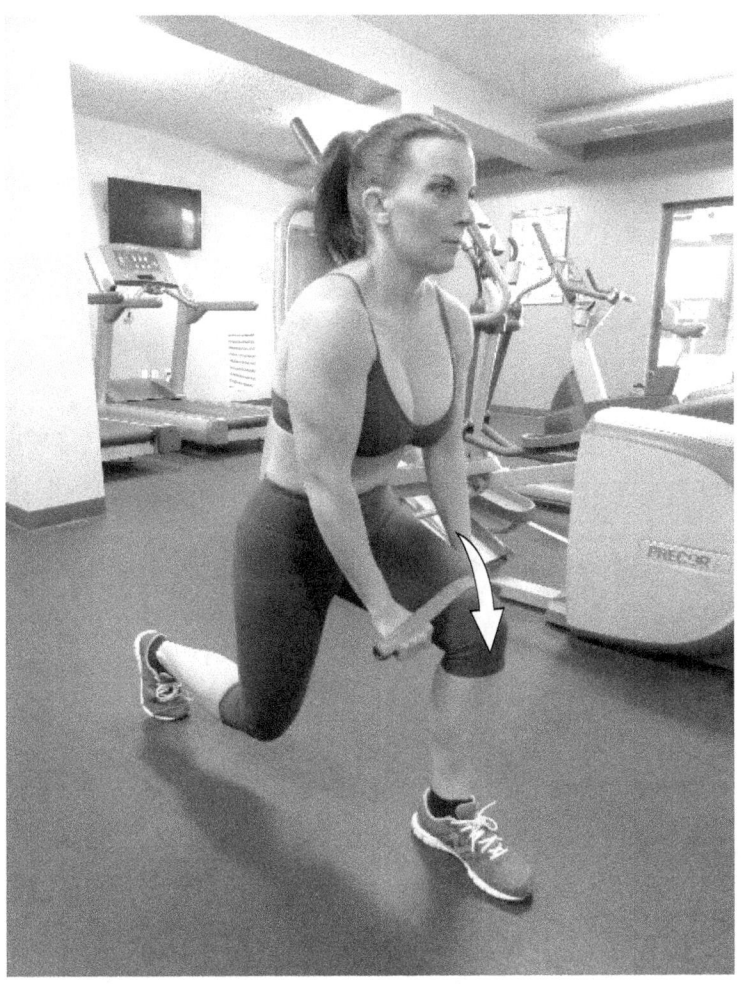

BONUS LEG EXERCISES

You have now completed the SSASS™ Workout! After 60 seconds of intense isometric exercise, your legs may feel a little wobbly.

If you feel like you have had enough, you can stop right here. If you would like to do two more exercises, continue to the next page! It is only another 20 seconds - right?!?!

ADDUCTOR

Sit on the floor in a bent-knee position, wrap two Iso-Bows® together to make a four-handle pair, and place them between the knees.

Squeeze the knees together to engage the inner thigh muscles.

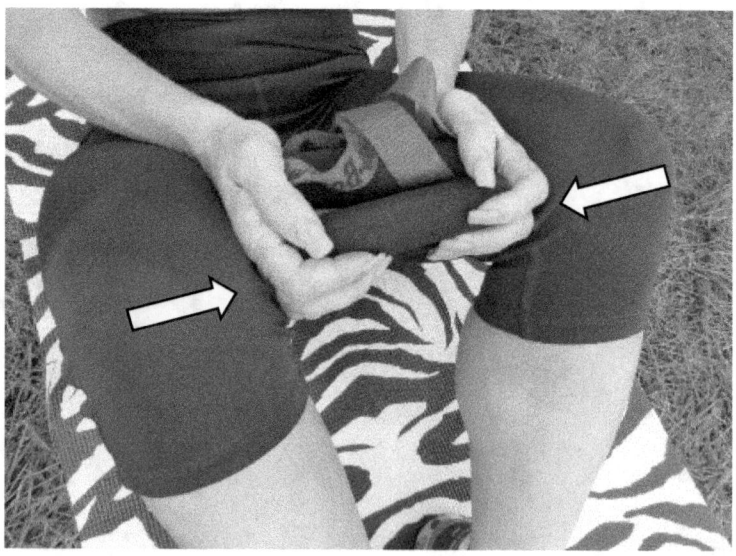

Breathe naturally and deeply in and out for about 10 full breaths, which will take about 1 second per breath.

Aim to perform an exercise breathing count of no less than 7 seconds and no longer than 10 seconds.

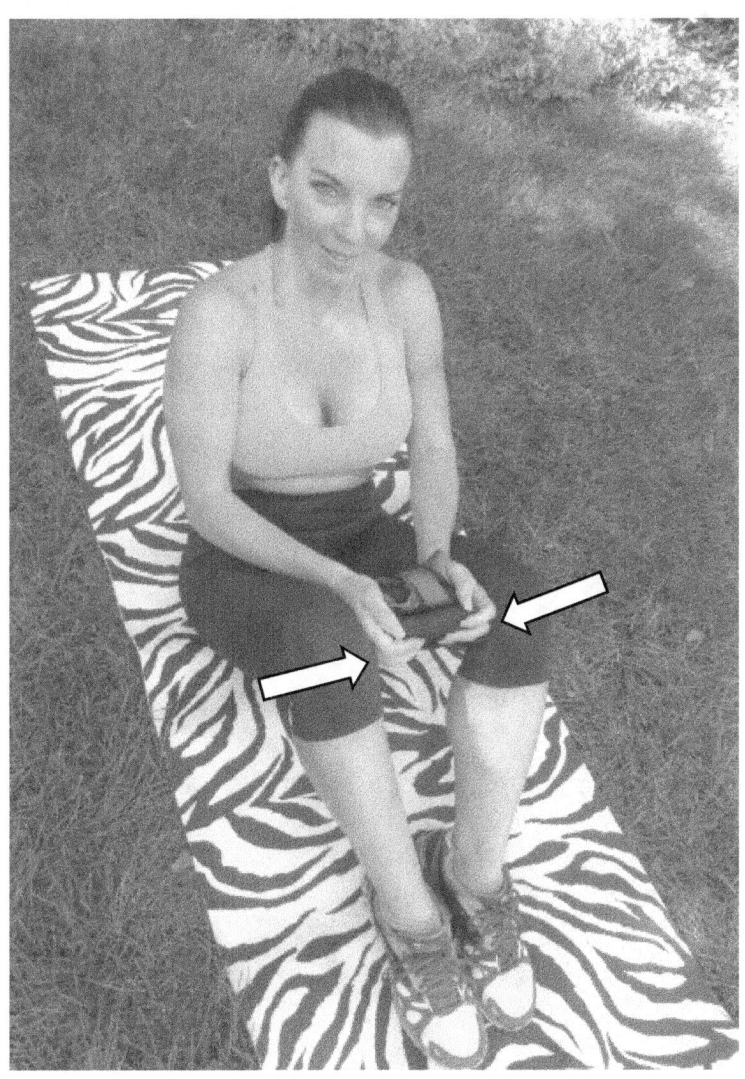

ABDUCTOR

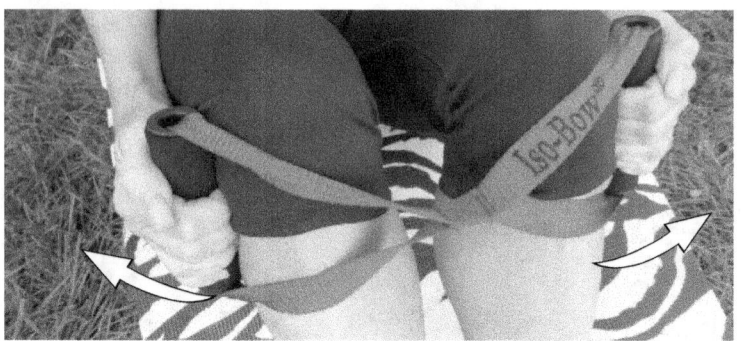

Sit on the floor in a bent-knee position, place the Iso-Bow® comfortably across the knees as shown and hold each handle firmly to prevent any movement from taking place. Pull your knees and legs apart sideways to engage the outer thigh, hip, and glute muscles. Breathe naturally and deeply in and out for about 10 full breaths, which will take about 1 second per breath. Aim to perform an exercise breathing count of no less than 7 seconds and no longer than 10 seconds.

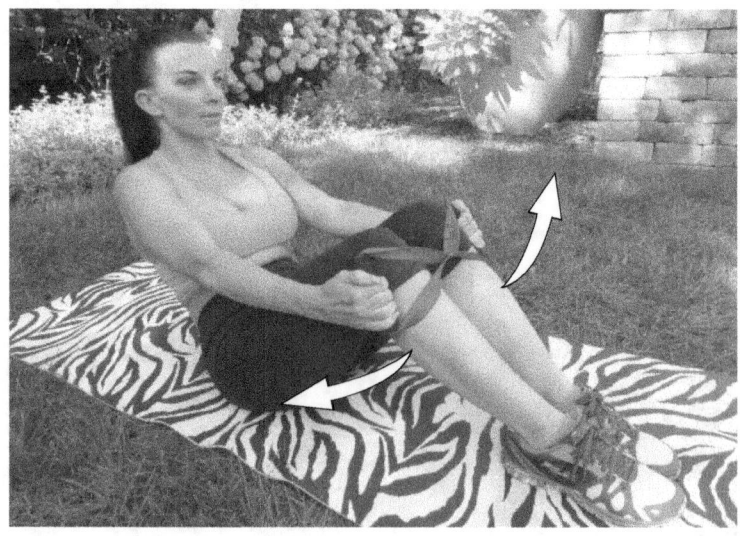

Chapter 9: INTERMEDIATE SSASS™ WORKOUT

Perform only one 7-second isometric exercise contraction.

▲ Before you begin the full isometric contraction part of the exercise, take between 2 and 3 additional seconds to perform Dynamic Flexation™ to help you properly engage the muscles and joints. Similarly, at the end of each isometric exercise, do the same in reverse as you disengage from the exercise over between 2 and 3 seconds.

INTERMEDIATE SQUAT

To perform the intermediate squat, stand shoulder-width apart with your feet.

Bend your knees as far as you are comfortably able to, bending only from the hips and keeping your back straight.

Hold both handles of an Iso-Bow® and extend your arms straight out in front of you to help you maintain balance.

Breathe naturally and deeply in and out for about 10 full breaths, which will take about 1 second per breath.

Aim to perform an exercise breathing count of no less than 7 seconds and no longer than 10 seconds.

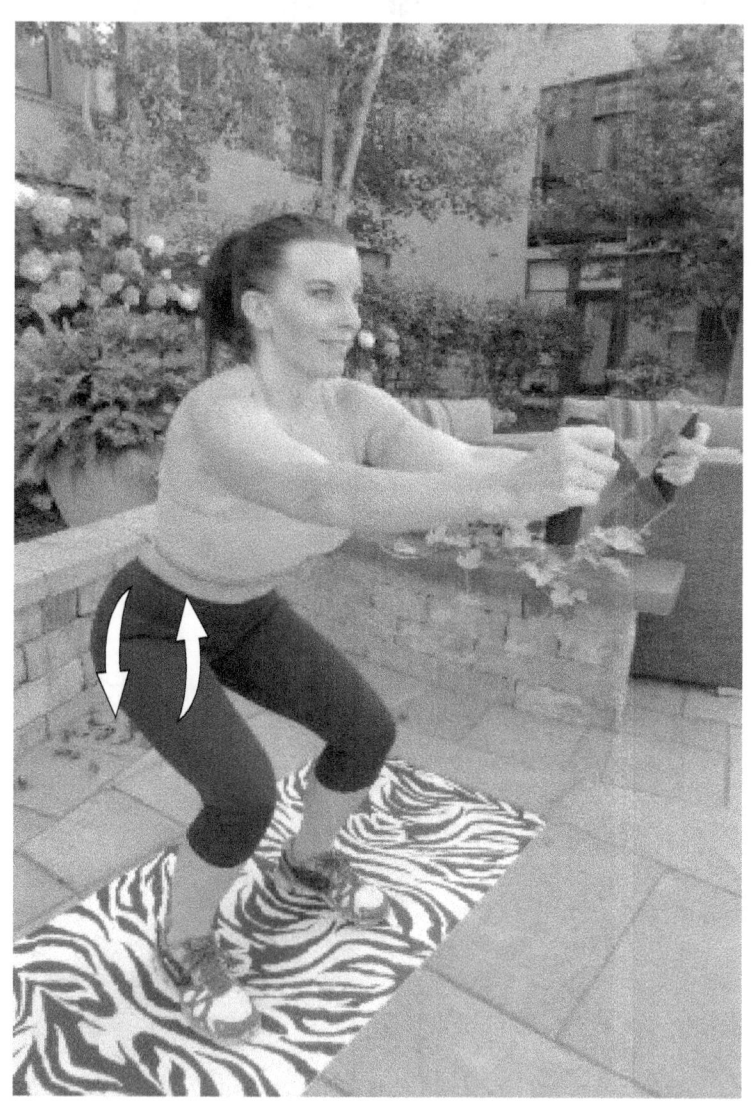

BENT LEG DEADLIFT

Place the loop handle of both Iso-Bows® around each foot as shown. Hold each handle firmly while maintaining a perfect bent-knee, semi-squat position with your back straight at all times, then attempt to stand up straight slowly.

Engage the muscles of the glutes, hamstrings, lower back, thighs, and other core muscles while the Iso-Bows® are secured by your feet, preventing movement.

Breathe naturally and deeply in and out for about 10 full breaths, which will take about 1 second per breath.

Aim to perform an exercise breathing count of no less than 7 seconds and no longer than 10 seconds.

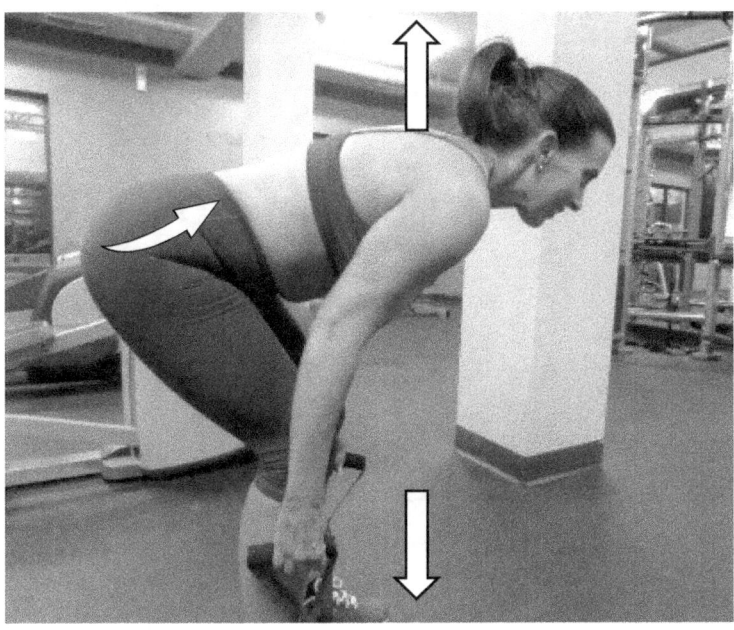

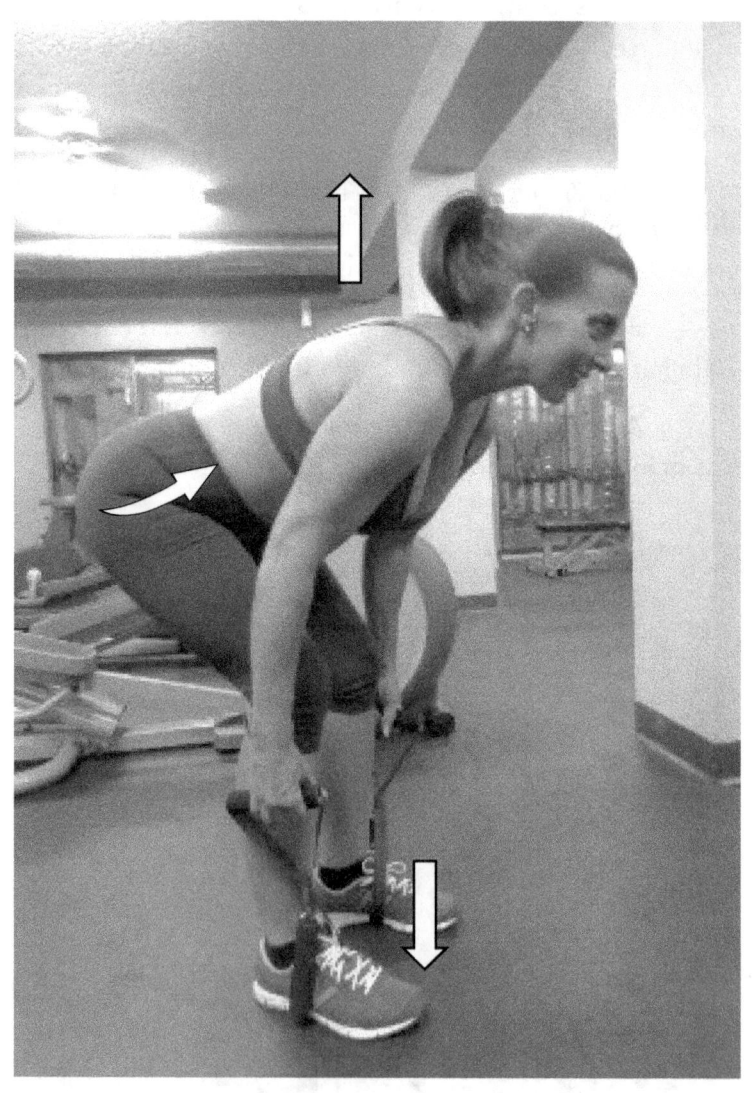

INTERMEDIATE SIDE LEG LUNGE – LEFT AND RIGHT LEG

Bend one knee out to one side at about a 90-degree angle to create a side leg lunge position. Hold an Iso-Bow® and comfortably place it around the upper shin, close to the knee of the bent leg.

You can use this position to provide extra resistance by pulling against it as you attempt to return to a standing position, holding the resistance in a mid-point leg lunge/split squat position.

Breathe naturally and deeply in and out for about 10 full breaths, which will take about 1 second per breath. Aim to perform an exercise breathing count of no less than 7 seconds and no longer than 10 seconds.   Repeat the same exercise with the other leg.

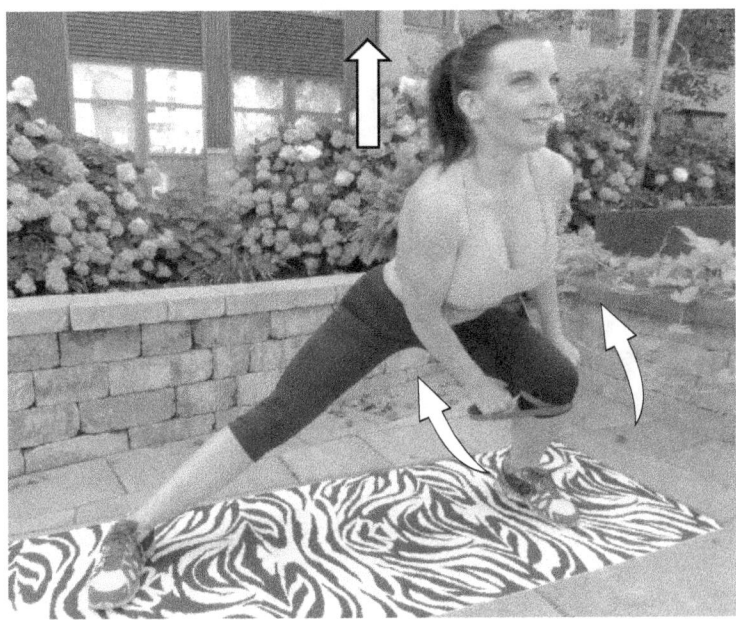

INTERMEDIATE FORWARD SPLIT SQUAT – LEFT AND RIGHT LEG

To perform the intermediate split squat, stand with your feet shoulder-width apart. Bend one knee forward to about 90 degrees while at the same time moving the other leg backwards, with your trailing knee close to the floor, to create a split squat position. Hold an Iso-Bow® and place it comfortably around the upper shin, close to the knee of the extended leg. You can use this position to provide extra resistance by pulling against it as you try to return to the standing position and hold the mid-point split squat position.

Breathe naturally and deeply in and out for about 10 full breaths, which will take about 1 second per breath. Aim to perform an exercise breathing count of no less than 7 seconds and no longer than 10 seconds. Repeat the same exercise with the other leg.

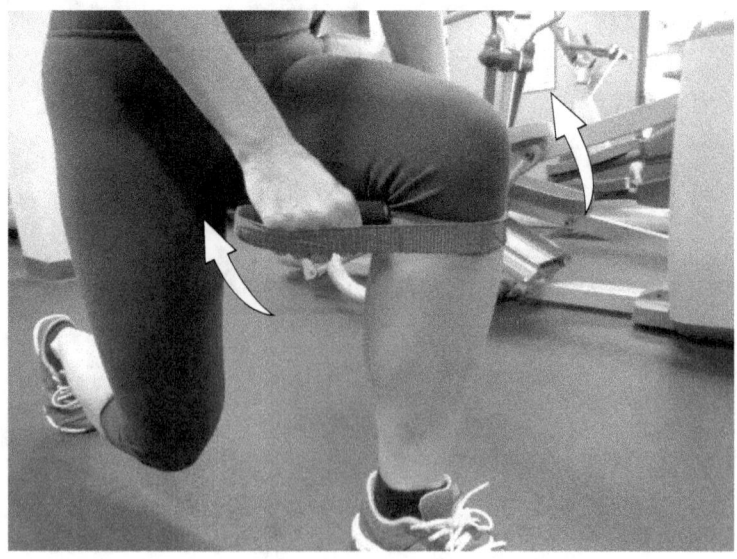

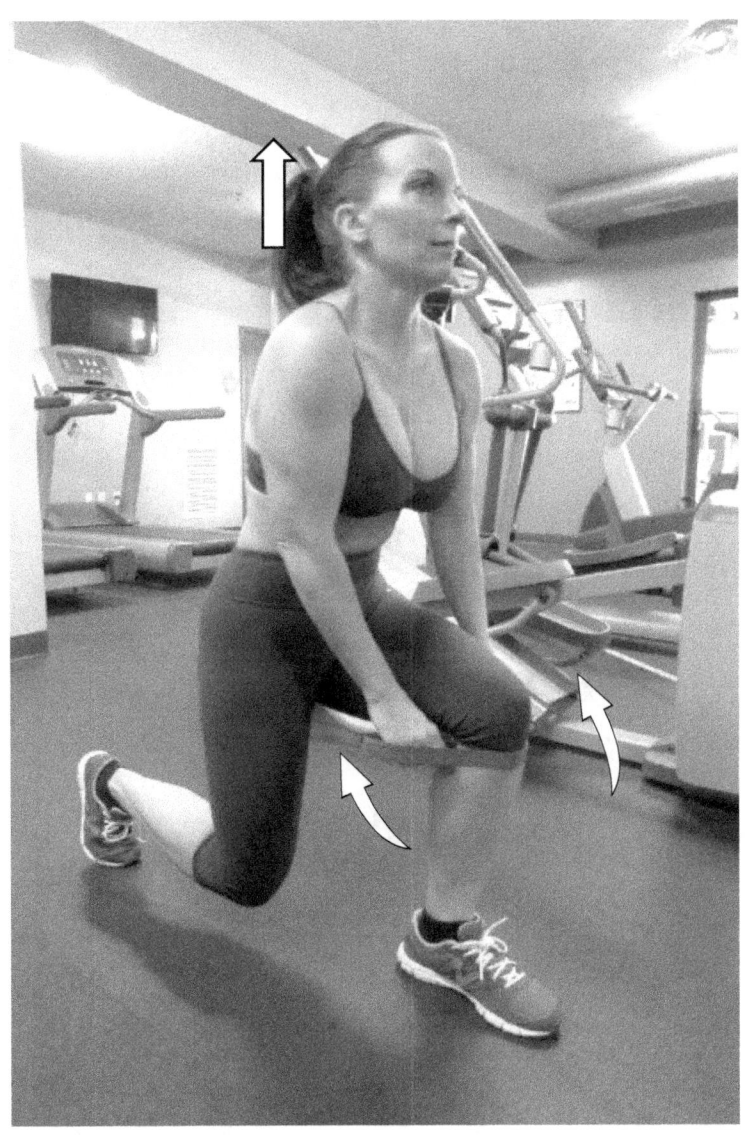

BONUS LEG EXERCISES

You have now completed the SSASS™ Workout! After 60 seconds of intense isometric exercise, your legs may feel a little wobbly.

If you feel like you have had enough, you can stop right here. If you would like to do two more exercises, continue to the next page! It is only another 20 seconds - right?!?!

ADDUCTOR

Sit on the floor in a bent-knee position, wrap two Iso-Bows® together to make a four-handle pair, and place them between the knees.

Squeeze the knees together to engage the inner thigh muscles.

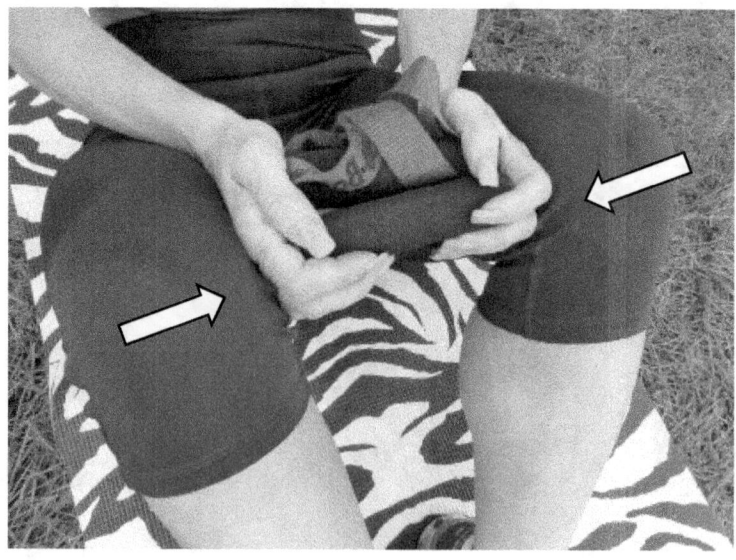

Breathe naturally and deeply in and out for about 10 full breaths, which will take about 1 second per breath.

Aim to perform an exercise breathing count of no less than 7 seconds and no longer than 10 seconds.

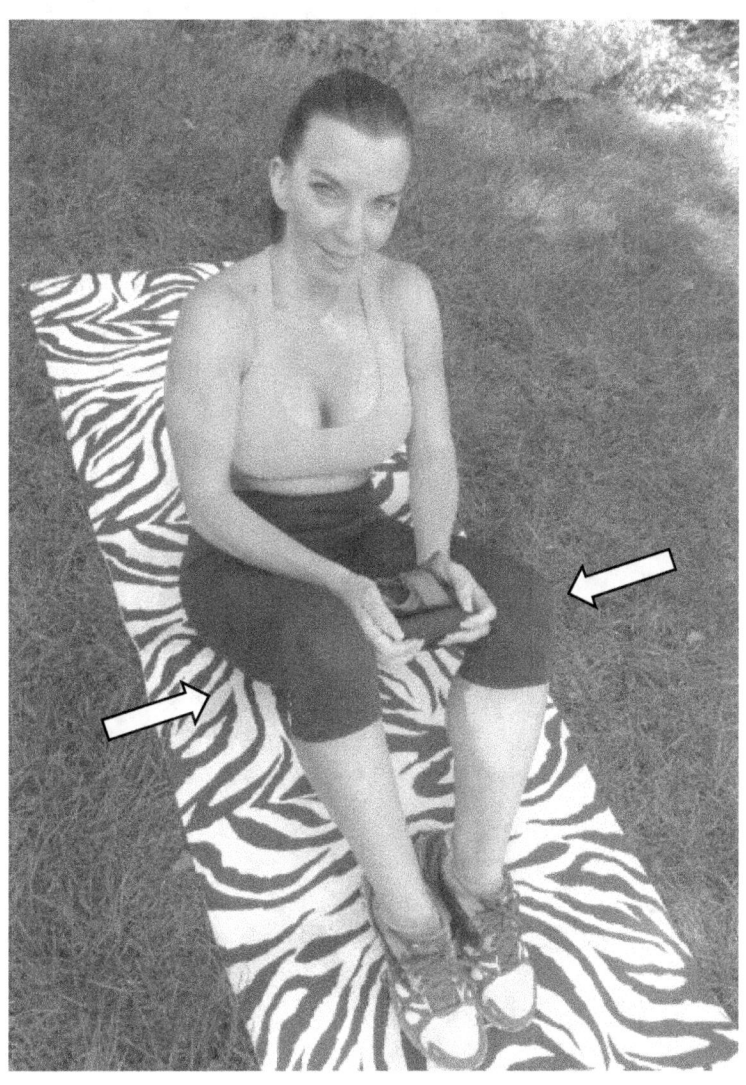

ABDUCTOR

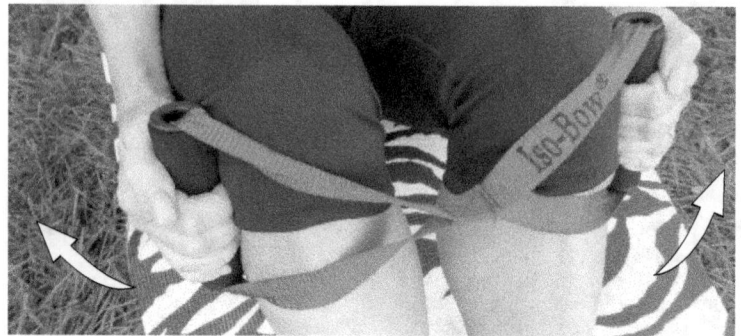

Sit on the floor in a bent-knee position, place the Iso-Bow® comfortably across the knees as shown and hold each handle firmly to prevent any movement from taking place. Pull your knees and legs apart sideways to engage the outer thigh, hip, and glute muscles. Breathe naturally and deeply in and out for about 10 full breaths, which will take about 1 second per breath. Aim to perform an exercise breathing count of no less than 7 seconds and no longer than 10 seconds.

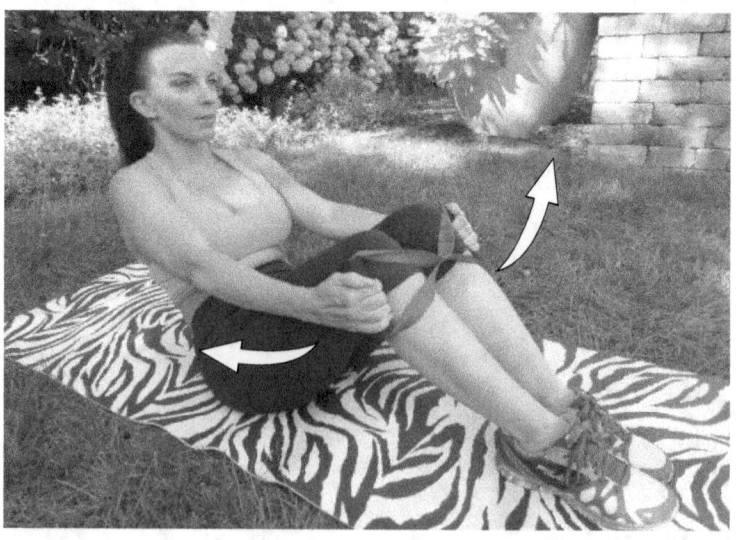

Chapter 10: ADVANCED
SSASS™ WORKOUT

Perform only one 7-second isometric exercise contraction.

⚠ Before you begin the full isometric contraction part of the exercise, take between 2 and 3 additional seconds to perform Dynamic Flexation™ to help you properly engage the muscles and joints. Similarly, at the end of each isometric exercise, do the same in reverse as you disengage from the exercise over between 2 and 3 seconds.

⚠ Perform the workout every day, taking weekends off or every other day, alternating with the 70 Second Difference Workout.

⚠ Take two days of rest over the weekend before starting the workout routine again on the following Monday.

ADVANCED SQUAT

Place the looped handle side of each Iso-Bow® around each foot as shown. Bend your knees deeply to assume the squat position, bending your torso only at the hips and keeping your back straight and upright at all times.

Grip each Iso-Bow® handle firmly and attempt to stand up straight by engaging your upper thigh and glute muscles. Naturally, you will not be able to move, but continue your attempt to stand up while maintaining the perfect mid-squat position as you do. Breathe naturally and deeply in and out for about 10 full breaths, which will take about 1 second per breath. Aim to perform an exercise breathing count of no less than 7 seconds and no longer than 10 seconds.

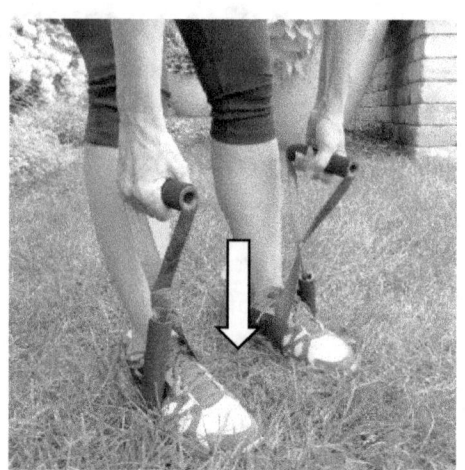

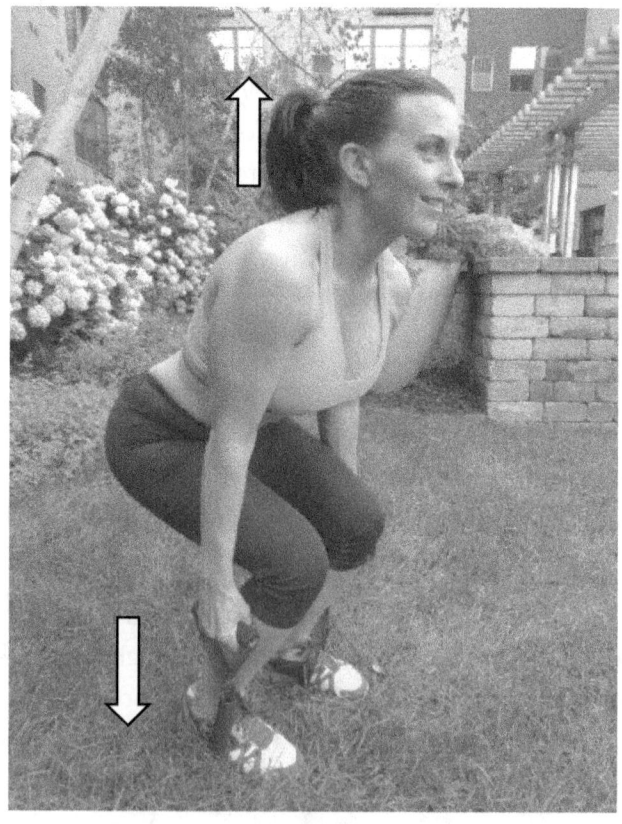

STRAIGHT LEG DEADLIFT

Place the loop of both Iso-Bows® around each foot as shown. Grip the handles firmly, bending over from the hips, with your knees only very slightly bent and your back straight at all times, then slowly attempt to stand up straight. Engage the muscles of the glutes, hamstrings, lower back, thighs, and other core muscles while the Iso-Bows® secured by your feet will prevent any movement from taking place. Breathe naturally and deeply in and out for about 10 full breaths, which will take about 1 second per breath. Aim to perform an exercise breathing count of no less than 7 seconds and no longer than 10 seconds.

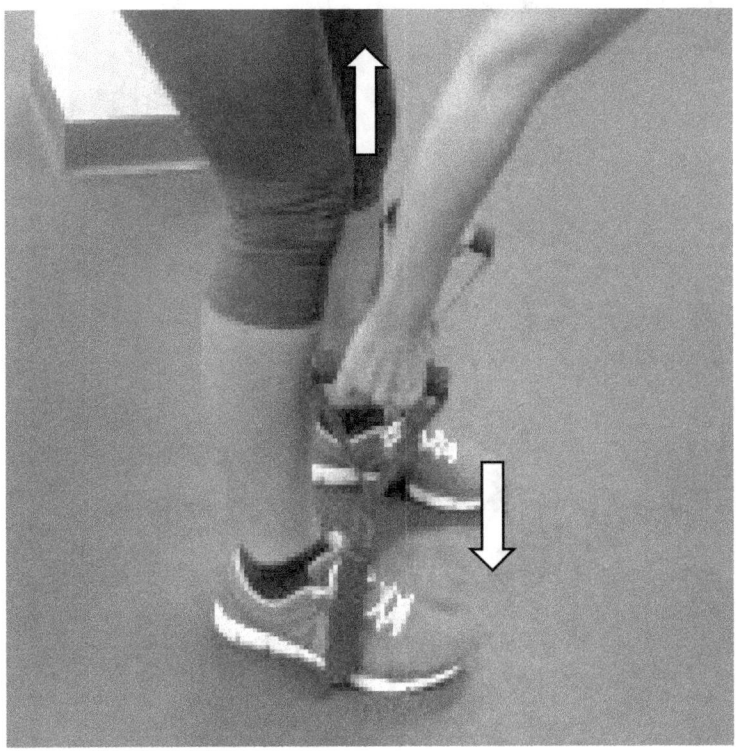

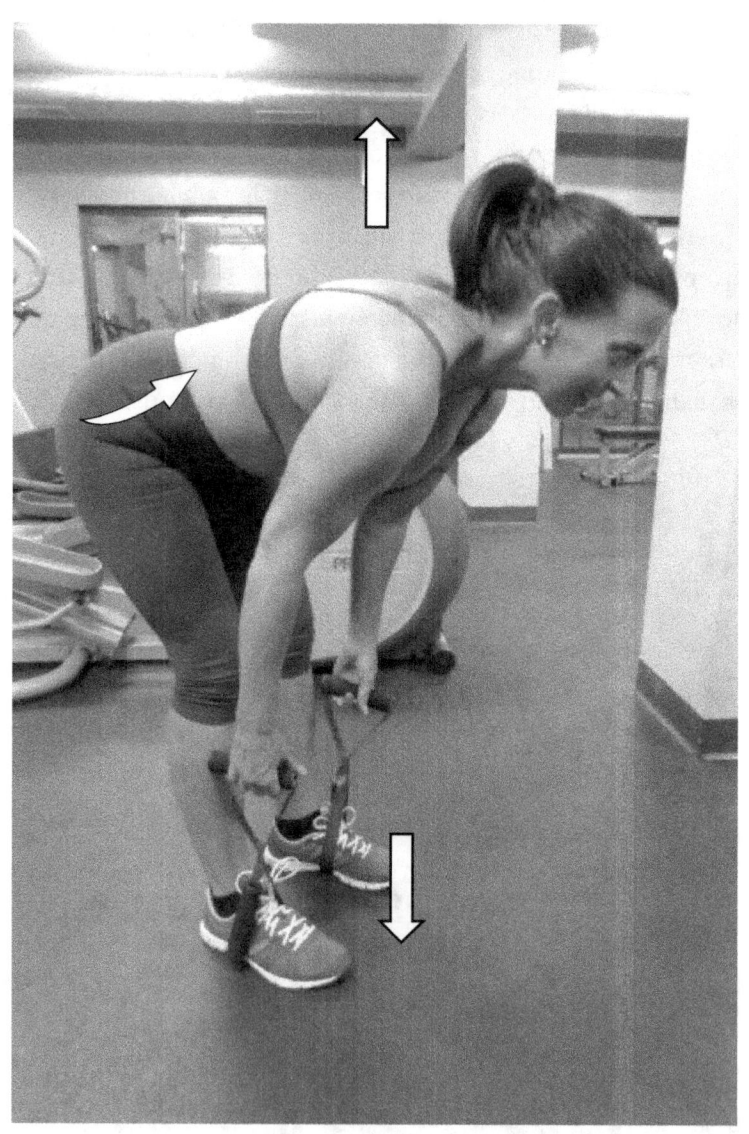

ADVANCED SIDE LEG LUNGE –
LEFT AND RIGHT SIDE

Place the looped ends of two Iso-Bows® around the foot as shown to make a double stirrup. Bend the knee of that leg to about 90 degrees while at the same time moving the other leg out sideways to create a side leg-lunge position. Hold both Iso-Bow® handles firmly, and keep your body upright and your back straight. Use and engage your leading leg's thigh and glute muscles as you attempt to straighten it and push upwards. Breathe naturally and deeply in and out for about 10 full breaths, which will take about 1 second per breath. Aim to perform an exercise breathing count of no less than 7 seconds and no longer than 10 seconds. Repeat the exercise with the other leg.

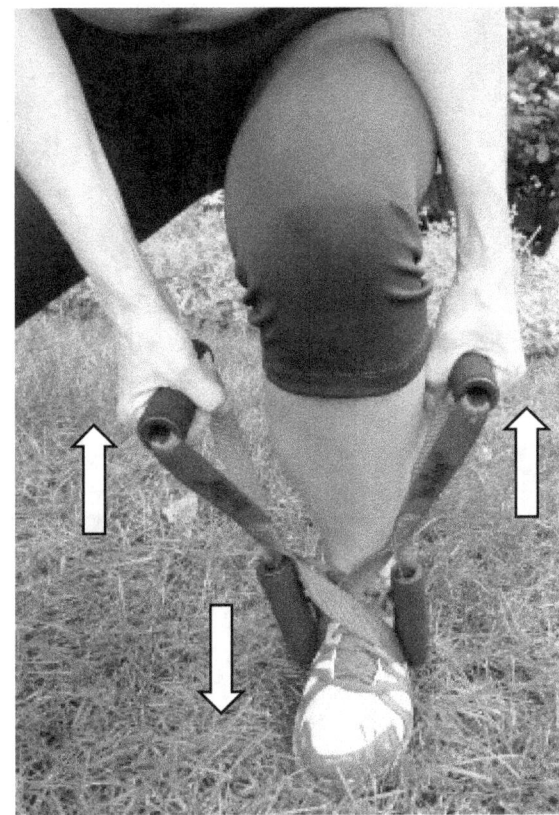

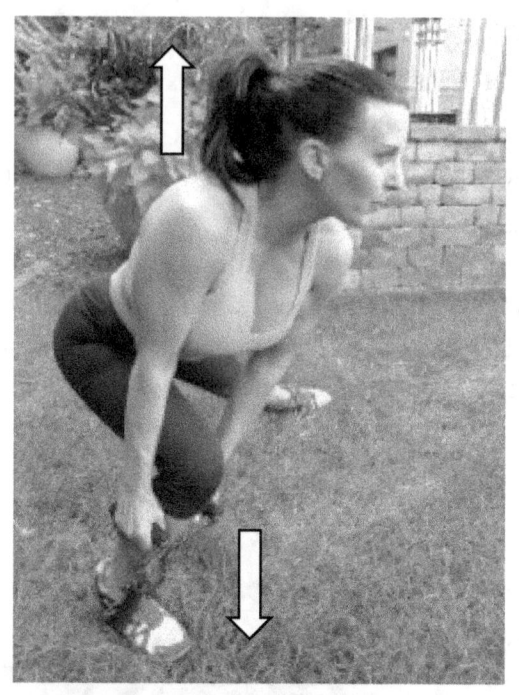

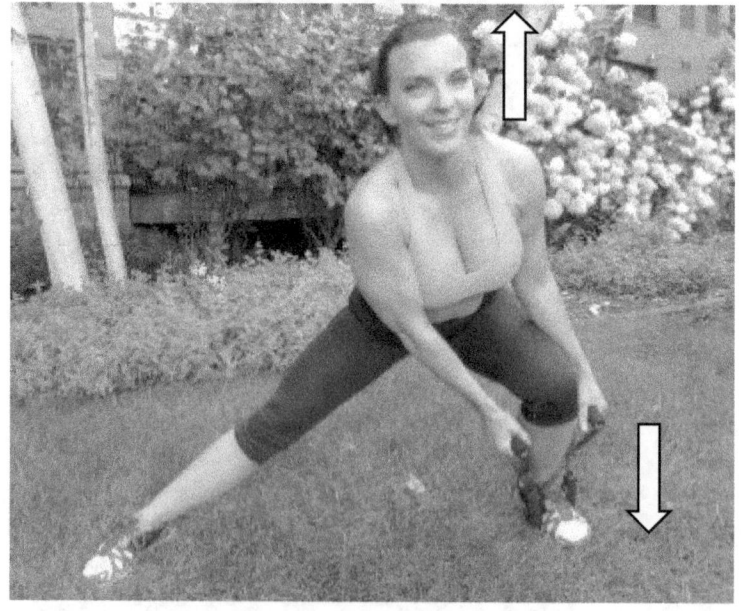

ADVANCED FORWARD SPLIT SQUAT

Place the looped ends of two Iso-Bows® around the foot as shown to make a double stirrup. Bend the knee to about 90 degrees while at the same time moving the other leg backwards, with your trailing knee close to the floor, to create a split squat position. Hold both Iso-Bow® handles firmly, and keep your body upright and your back straight. Use and engage your leading leg's thigh and glute muscles as you attempt to straighten it and push upwards.

Breathe naturally and deeply in and out for about 10 full breaths, which will take about 1 second per breath. Aim to perform an exercise breathing count of no less than 7 seconds and no longer than 10 seconds. Repeat the exercise with the other leg.

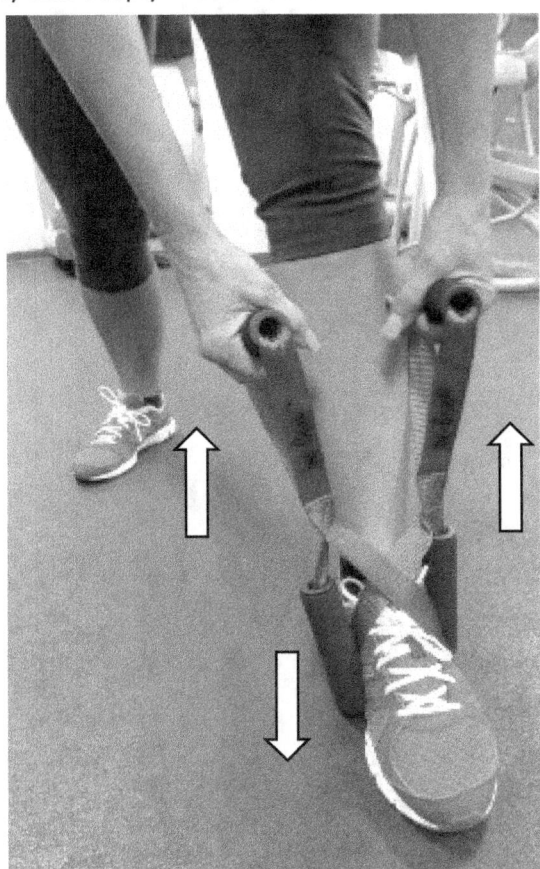

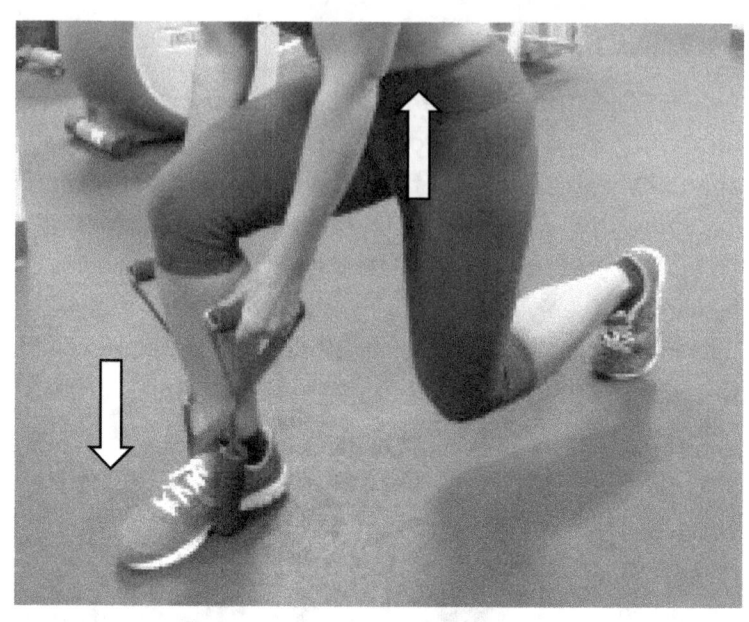

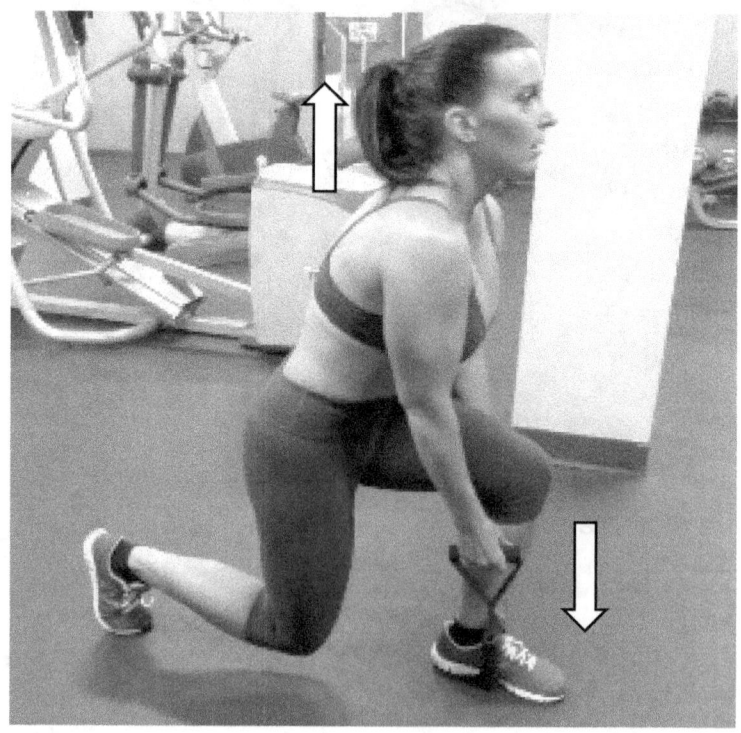

BONUS LEG EXERCISES

You have now completed the SSASS™ Workout! After 60 seconds of intense isometric exercise, your legs may feel wobbly.

If you feel like you have had enough, you can stop right here. If you would like to do two more exercises, continue to the next page! It is only another 20 seconds - right?!?!

ADDUCTOR

Sit on the floor in a bent-knee position, wrap two Iso-Bows® together to make a four-handle pair, and place them between the knees.

Squeeze the knees together to engage the inner thigh muscles.

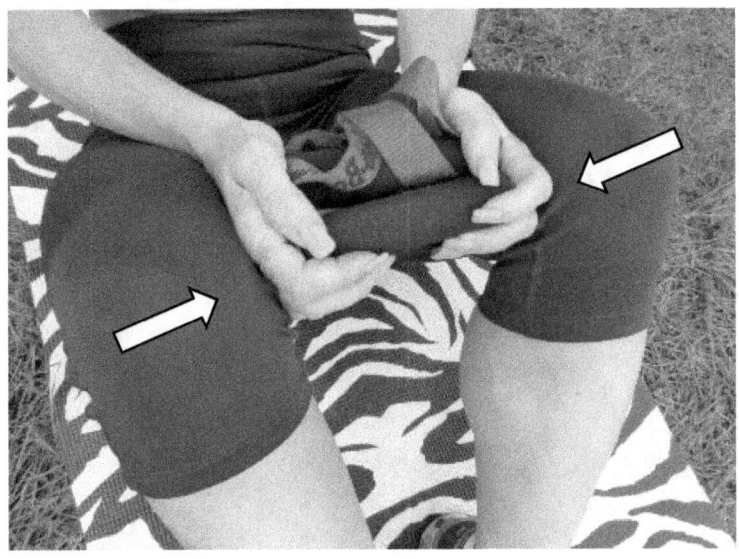

Breathe naturally and deeply in and out for about 10 full breaths, which will take about 1 second per breath.

Aim to perform an exercise breathing count of no less than 7 seconds and no longer than 10 seconds.

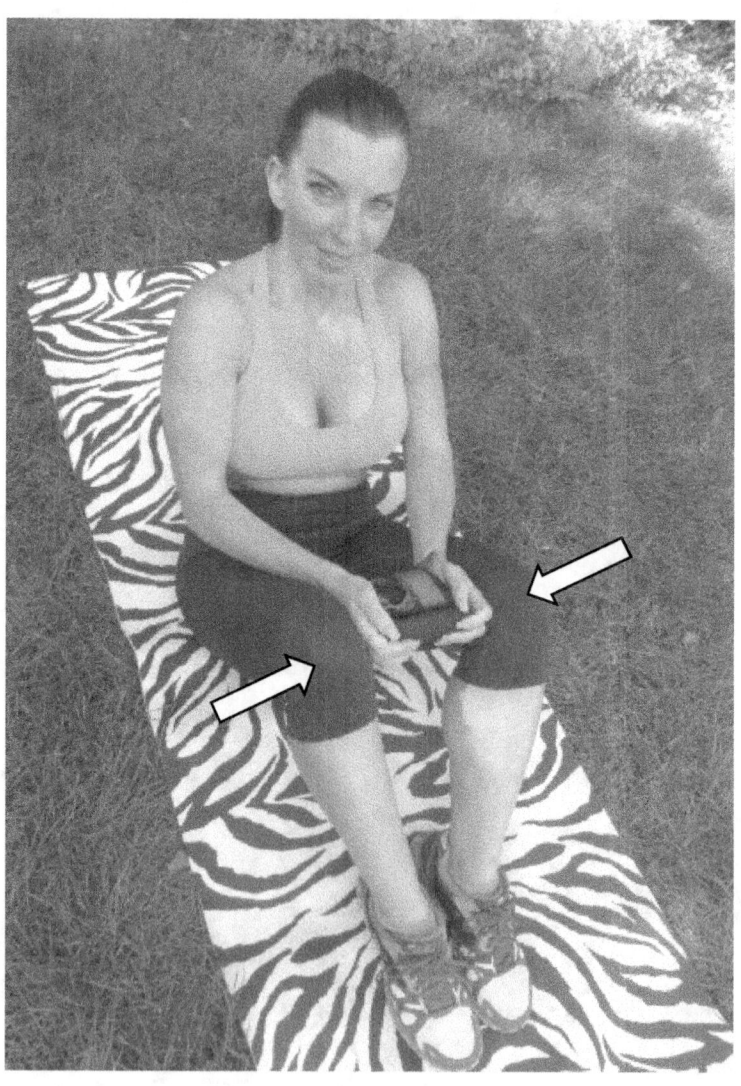

ABDUCTOR

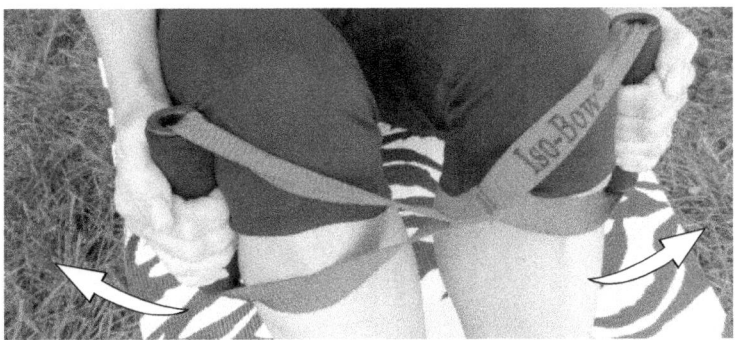

Sit on the floor in a bent-knee position, place the Iso-Bow® comfortably across the knees as shown and hold each handle firmly to prevent any movement from taking place. Pull your knees and legs apart sideways to engage the outer thigh, hip, and glute muscles. Breathe naturally and deeply in and out for about 10 full breaths, which will take about 1 second per breath. Aim to perform an exercise breathing count of no less than 7 seconds and no longer than 10 seconds.

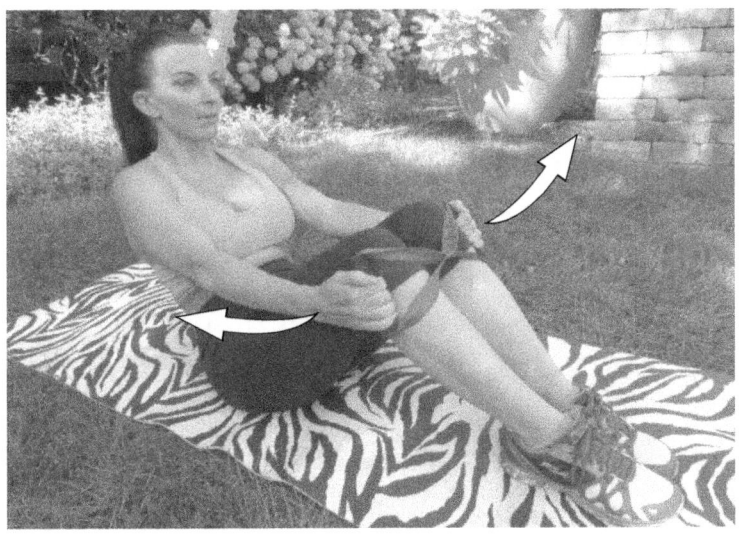

Chapter 11: Conclusion

When you eventually read this section as a natural progression after performing the entire SSASS™ Workout daily for a few weeks, you will have a firmer, tighter, and lifted rear end. We recommend you keep doing the exercises, and you will continually notice that you are stronger and fitter than before.

Many people will have made an excellent start on a much longer journey, which is needed as they completely overhaul the size and shape of their bodies. Other people will have already forged the new body size, strength and shape they have always wanted.

I hope you have enjoyed learning the three different SSASS™ Workout routines. Feel free to mix them up and do what is most comfortable for you. It is also a good idea to look at our other ISOfitness™ courses and fitness routines to learn some of the upper-body exercises.

We highly recommend that everyone do exactly what Brian and I do now: always keep a pair of Iso-Bow® units with you, and USE THEM REGULARLY!

You can take the SSASS™ Workout or any of our other weekly workouts or courses and use them as a stand-alone daily or weekly exercise plan. Whatever your status and journey in this respect, we would like to sincerely thank you for performing The SSASS™ Workout and encourage you to make an ISOfitness™ workout an integral part of your daily life.

Exercise boredom is NOT an option with the ISOfitness™ exercise system. Our growing library of exercises will help keep your sessions varied, interesting, and exciting, ensuring your success in fitness, body shaping, and strength!

What is ISOfitness™?

The ISOfitness™ exercise system is simply our general name for applied isometric exercises. These include isometric, isokinetic, and combined isotonic exercises, advanced isometric exercise techniques, Dynamic Flexation™, Super-Slow Isotonic Flexation™, and the newly proven science of USB-UHT™ (Ultra Short Burst – Ultra High Intensity) exercises. It also includes our own hybrid TRISOmetric™ exercise system.

What is TWiEA™?

TWiEA™ is the acronym for The World Isometric Exercise Association. Its mission is to help set and maintain standards of excellence in teaching and promoting all types of isometric exercise. It seeks to ensure that scientifically proven isometric exercise techniques are taught as part of an integrated total-body exercise solution provided by fitness professionals. This increases the probability that busy clients facing real-life time crunches can maintain an effective exercise program. Isometric exercise is every bit as effective at building muscle and strength as other traditional forms of resistance training. It is also a time— and money-saving exercise solution that almost anyone can perform without any special equipment.

www.HelenRenee.com – www.BrianSterlingVete.com

113

Other books by Brian Sterling-Vete and Helen Renée Wuorio

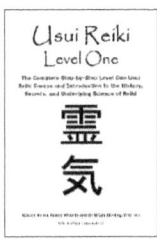

Usui Reiki Level One

An introduction to Reiki, covering its history and supporting science, is presented in an easy step-by-step format. This book and others in the series are course manuals for our online or in-person students.

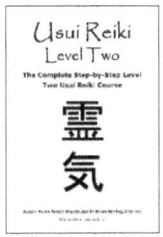

Usui Reiki Level Two

The Reiki Level Two course advances your journey, teaching Power Symbols and their usage. It excludes the history and science from book one and is structured logically in a clear, step-by-step format.

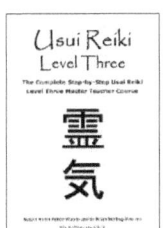

Usui Reiki Level Three

The Level Three Master Teacher course finalises the journey for Level Two practitioners. It focuses solely on Level Three concepts organised in a step-by-step format.

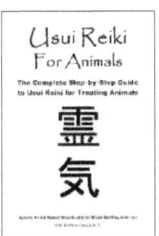

Usui Reiki Compendium (Levels One & Two)

The Reiki Compendium is a complete book of our Level One and Two courses, ideal for anyone wanting to progress through all levels of their Reiki Journey. It also serves as a manual for our students.

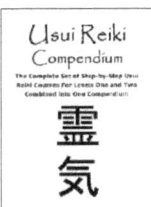

Usui Reiki for Treating Animals

This is perfect for practitioners of all levels wanting to learn safe and effective treatment technique, chakras and energy centres unique to specific animals.

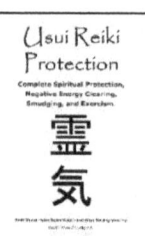

Usui Reiki Protection

The complete guide to spiritual protection, negative energy clearing, smudging, and exorcism, essential for every paranormal investigator and anyone wishing to clear people and places of negative energy.

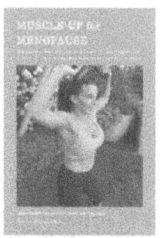

Muscle-up For Menopause

Menopause is inevitable, so take control. Brief, intense exercises with minimal recovery demands and a high-protein plant-based diet positively impact your menopause experience.

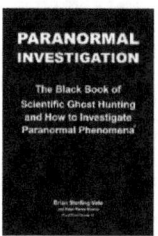

Paranormal Investigation - The Black Book of Scientific Ghost Hunting

It contains a scientific critical path graphic to work from and a step-by-step guide to a complete professional paranormal investigation.

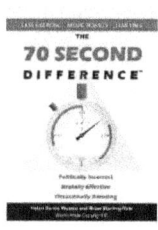

The 70 Second Difference - Politically Incorrect, Occasionally Amusing, and Brutally Effective

Just 70 seconds of focused science-based daily exercise can provide a total-body workout.

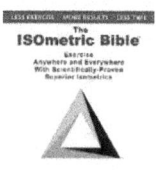

The ISOmetric Bible - Exercise Anywhere with Scientifically Proven Isometrics

A complete, scientific, and user-friendly benchmark book about scientifically proven isometric exercises: no special equipment is needed for a total-body workout.

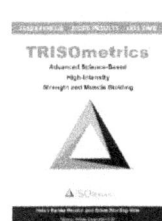

TRISOmetrics - Advanced Science-Based High-Intensity Strength and Muscle Building
This advanced, high-intensity exercise system combines three proven techniques into a powerful new approach, with or without equipment, while travelling or in the gym.

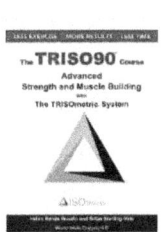

The TRISO90 Course – Advanced Strength and Muscle Building with TRISOmetrics.
A 90-day step-by-step advanced bodybuilding and strength-training course performed with or without equipment or in a gym routine.

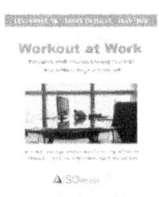

Workout at Work - Exercise at Work Without Anyone Even Knowing What You're Doing!
Science-based Isometric exercises let you work out effectively and discreetly without leaving your desk.

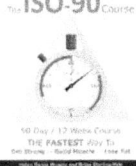

The ISO90 Course – The 12-Week/90-Day Shape-up and Get Strong Course. A complete step-by-step 90-day isometric body shaping, bodybuilding, and strength-building course is ideal for both beginners and advanced.

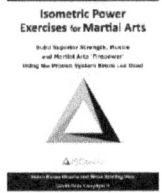

Isometric Power Exercises for Martial Arts - Build Superior Strength, Muscle and Martial Arts 'Firepower' Using the Proven System Bruce Lee Used. This is a valuable resource for practical isometric exercises that build serious strength, muscle, and martial arts firepower.

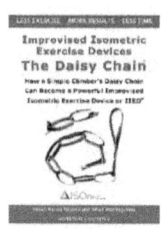

Improvised Isometric Exercise Devices (IIEDs) - The Daisy Chain

This is a resource for practical exercises that can be performed and for learning how to extend the daisy chain safely.

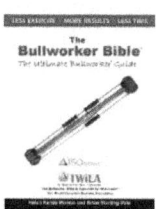

Improvised Isometric Exercise Devices (IIEDs) - The Climber's Sling

This valuable resource lists practical isometric exercises that can be performed and how to safely extend the climber's sling.

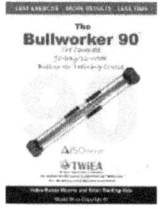

The Bullworker Bible - The Ultimate Science-Based Guide to The Classic Personal Multi-Gym. Approved by Bullworker.com. It is a complete, science-based user-friendly book and companion to The Bullworker 90 Course.

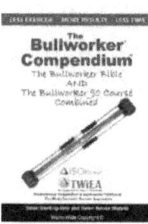

The Bullworker 90™ Course - The Ultimate Science-Based 12-Week/90-Day Get Strong and Grow Muscle Course Approved by The Bullworker makers, this complete 90-day course and companion book to The Bullworker Bible.

The Bullworker Compendium - The Bullworker Bible and The Bullworker90 Course Combined

Approved by the makers of The Bullworker. The Bullworker Compendium™ combines both The Bullworker Bible™ and The Bullworker 90™ Course in a single huge book.

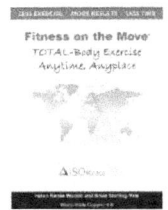

Fitness on the Move

Practical exercises that can be performed while travelling almost anywhere, even in a vehicle. If there is enough space to sit and stand, you can have a total-body workout!

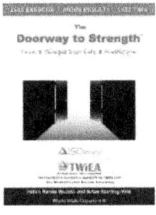

The Doorway to Strength - Turn a Door into a Strength-Building Multigym. It shows how a simple door, doorway, and frame can create a multi-gym of exercises using the amazing Iso-Bow®. Required: 2 x Iso-Bows®, a solid door and frame, and a door wedge/stop.

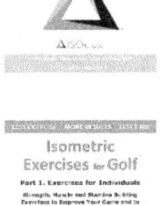

Feel Better In 70 Seconds

Studies show that brief exercise combats depression without significant cost or time. Just 70 seconds of continuous movement allows a full-body workout using isometric exercises, requiring 2 x Iso-Bows®.

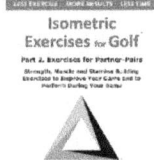

Isometric Exercises for Golf Part 1. Exercises for Individuals. Isometric exercises can turn a round of golf into a full-body workout at each hole, using a golf club as a makeshift exercise tool. Part 1 provides customised exercises to improve swing power for individual needs.

Isometric Exercises for Golf Part 2. Partner-Pairs. The companion to Book 1 focuses on exercises best performed in partnered pairs during breaks, games, or practice sessions.

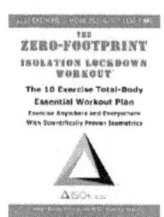

The Zero-Footprint Isolation Lockdown Workout. Ten essential total-body exercises can be done anywhere; if you can stand or sit, you can have a powerful workout in just 70 seconds a day!

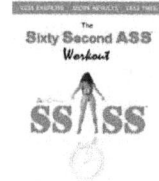

The Sixty Second ASS Workout - Shape, Tone, Lift, and Get the Backside You've Always Wanted. The fastest and most effective "ass" workout ever devised. Scientifically proven exercises deliver a no-nonsense, time-efficient workout.

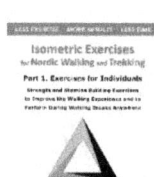

Isometric Exercises for Nordic Walking and Trekking - Part 1. Exercises for Individuals. Perform total-body isometric exercises during walk breaks using walking poles as an Improvised Isometric Exercise Device. Book 1 serves as a resource guide for individuals.

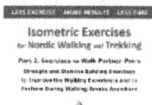
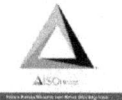

Isometric Exercises for Nordic Walking and Trekking - Part 2. Exercises for Walk Partner-Pairs.
This is the companion to Book 1, focusing on exercises performed as a walking partner.

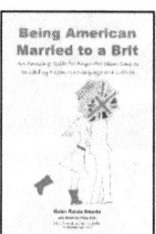

Being American Married to a Brit - An Amusing Guide for Anglo-American Couples. This quirky, fun-filled roller coaster ride is about how even the most basic everyday transatlantic conversations can bring laughter. It's dedicated to all transatlantic couples.

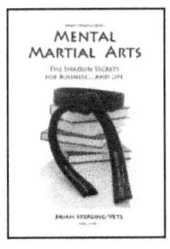

Mental Martial Arts - Intellectual Life and Business Combat Skills. An intellectual language and combat skills system based on martial arts principles. Learn to guide and redirect the energy of influential individuals and large organisations to achieve goals.

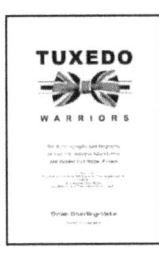

Tuxedo Warriors
The companion book to The Tuxedo Warrior expands on the story, serving as both a biography and autobiography of cult author Cliff Twemlow. It also includes unique insights from Brian Sterling-Vete.

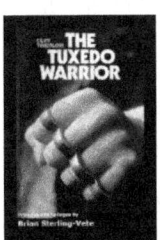

The Tuxedo Warrior by Cliff Twemlow – A doorman manages respect using either diplomacy or force. This requires balancing peaceful solutions with violent encounters, providing a raw perspective on the lively yet perilous world of clubland peacekeeping.

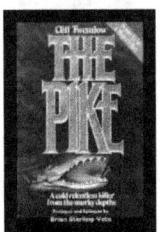

The Pike by Cliff Twemlow – A monstrous pike terrorises Lake Windermere, attacking people and boats, causing panic. Some exploit the chaos, hindering the creature's capture to profit as the terror escalates.

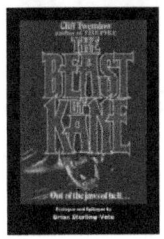

The Beast of Kane by Cliff Twemlow – The Gordon family invites darkness by adopting a stray Elkhound, igniting ancient evil prophecies. Kane faces supernatural terror, from animal attacks to gruesome murder, as a chilling winter amplifies the fear in town.

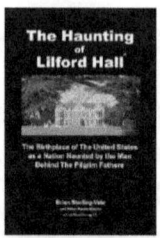

The Haunting of Lilford Hall - The Birthplace of the United States as a Nation Haunted by the Man Behind The Pilgrim Fathers.
A baffling case of paranormal activity occurred from 2012 to 2013, involving multiple people.

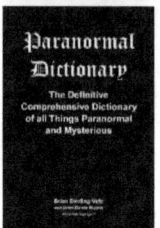

Paranormal Dictionary
This comprehensive guide covers the most common paranormal terminology, entities, and equipment used during investigations. Ideal for both new and experienced investigators.

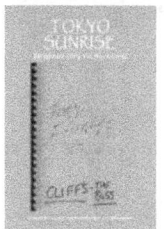

Tokyo Sunrise Background Story and Script
One of Cliff Twemlow's famous film concepts. Cinematographer Robert Foster produced a promotional sizzle reel, aiming to sell the movie to potential investors. This also tells the story of the Richard Gere connection.

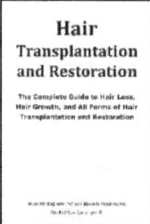

Hair Transplantation and Restoration
The essential guide to hair loss, growth, and ALL forms of hair transplantation and restoration. Malcolm Mendelsohn is the world's #1 independent expert with almost 50 years of experience.

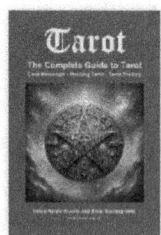

Tarot – The Complete Guide
Explore the ultimate tarot guide, covering its history, card styles, and meanings. Master the art and science of tarot reading with insights and secret techniques from an internationally acclaimed Tarot Master, Helen Renée.

Tarot Card Spreads

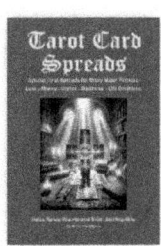

Discover the ultimate tarot spread guide, featuring various spreads for love, money, career, business, and key life decisions. It includes detailed diagrams and descriptions to enhance your tarot practice.

Quantum Paranormal

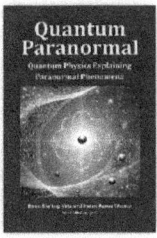

Quantum physics meets the paranormal, offering fascinating explanations about the existence of paranormal phenomena and the mechanisms underpinning them. This deeply controversial book also challenges a crucial belief at the foundation of the Christian Church.

www.ingramcontent.com/pod-product-compliance
Lightning Source LLC
Chambersburg PA
CBHW072202280526
45788CB00002B/837